Social and Cognitive Pharmacy

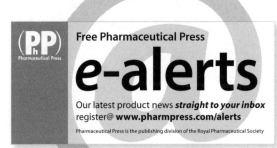

Social and Cognitive Pharmacy

Theory and case studies

Parastou Donyai PhD, BPharm(Hons), MRPharmS, PGDPRM(Open), PGCertLTHE, PGCertEBP

Pharmacist

Lecturer, Pharmacy Practice, Reading School of Pharmacy

Whiteknights, Reading, Berkshire, UK

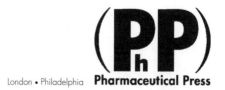

London • Philadelphia **Pharmaceutical Press**

Published by Pharmaceutical Press

1 Lambeth High Street, London SE1 7JN, UK
University City Science Center, Suite 5E, 3624 Market Street, Philadelphia,
PA 19104, USA

(**PP**) is a trade mark of Pharmaceutical Press
Pharmaceutical Press is the publishing division of the Royal Pharmaceutical
Society

First published 2012

Typeset by River Valley Technologies, India
Printed in Great Britain by TJ International, Padstow, Cornwall

ISBN 978 0 85369 899 9

'Solved riddles look easy'
Persian proverb

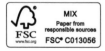

Contents

Foreword

Recognition of the value of patient-centred care is now embedded in health-care policy and in the principles espoused by healthcare practitioners. However, delivering patient-centred care may not always be intuitive. To date, much of the intellectual effort at understanding and delivering patient-centred care has been directed at medical colleagues, and pharmacists have been left to generalise from medical texts to their own professional context.

This book is an excellent overview of some key theories and concepts from health psychology and, to a lesser extent, sociology, presented in a practical format that will be of great value in helping pharmacists optimise their professional patient-centred interactions with patients and consumers. The important and often complex theoretical sections are integrated well with practical pharmacy-related examples, which should allow readers to conceptualise some of the abstract ideas presented in the pharmacy context, and thereby give them a useful in-depth understanding of how a theoretical approach to analysing, interpreting and managing different types of inter-actions could help them maximise the impact of their own knowledge for the benefit of the patient/consumer. Although the book is largely directed at an undergraduate readership, and has clear indications of what might be expected of students at different stages of the curriculum, it also could be regarded as an excellent primer for any pharmacist wanting to update their practice. For such readers, the case studies and self-assessment questions can also be used for reflection, and should facilitate the completion of continuing professional development records, and impart optimal benefit from the learning cycle.

In summary, this book logically presents some complex ideas sequentially, building to a comprehensive package of 'tools' to inform pharmacist-led, patient-centred care. Although most examples are based in community pharmacies, they are generic enough to be relevant to pharmacists working in any other patient-facing role, and also to those looking to explore their current practice systematically through research.

This book fills a critical gap in the pharmacy literature and is long overdue.

Professor Christine Bond
Chair in General Practice and Primary Care,
University of Aberdeen

Preface

The aim of this book is to provide undergraduate students of pharmacy, postgraduate pharmacists and university lecturers with a practical book for the teaching and learning of sociology and psychology, as applicable to pharmacy practice.

When this book was being written, the indicative syllabus for UK-accredited pharmacy degree courses (as set by the General Pharmaceutical Council) detailed the teaching and learning of specific areas, including principles and methodologies of the social and behavioural sciences relevant to pharmacy; health and illness: definitions and perceptions; the ideas and approaches of compliance or concordance in healthcare provision, particularly as they apply to taking medicines; the pharmacist's contribution to the promotion of good health and disease prevention; and social services' research methods and results relevant to pharmacy. At the point of going to press, the latest reworking of the indicative syllabus was included in *Standards for the Initial Education and Training of Pharmacists* (General Pharmaceutical Council, May 2011). These too emphasise the teaching of sociology and psychology, albeit under broader headings, so that, for example 'How people work' recommends teaching social and behavioural science, health psychology and behavioural medicine. These newer guidelines can be deemed as relatively unspecific, which means there is now an even greater need for a book that maps out sociological and psychological information with which to teach pharmacy students.

A survey published in the journal *Pharmacy Education* in 2006 (vol. 6, pages 125–131) revealed that 'social pharmacy' (the umbrella term for social and behavioural sciences relevant to pharmacy) was embedded in the MPharm curriculum of all the schools of pharmacy in the UK. The authors established that the introduction of social pharmacy into the curriculum and its subsequent organisation had been driven primarily by pharmacists rather than social scientists. Although pharmacy experience being brought to the teaching of social science was considered valuable, the authors thought this was not in itself adequate, nor was simply having an understanding of the methodological and theoretical principles underscoring social scientific enquiry. What was deemed important was the ability to provide content of immediate relevance to professional practice. Although there are textbooks available that cover some aspects of social and behavioural knowledge deemed relevant to pharmacy, none provide an easy-to-use medium for understanding how to apply the relevant psychosocial knowledge to everyday pharmacy issues. This book aims to elucidate the relationship between the principles, methodologies and theories of the social and behavioural sciences and their application to pharmacy practice to benefit students of pharmacy, postgraduate pharmacists and academics. Although the proposed readership is wide, the book's primary aim is to present concepts in as straightforward a manner as possible. More advanced readers can use the book with this proviso in mind.

This book demonstrates the relevance of sociology and psychology to pharmacy and provides both students, and lecturers who teach the subject, with an understanding of how to apply theory to professional practice. The chapters start with an introduction to sociology and psychology as individual disciplines. The main focus of the first chapter is to describe the importance of studying these disciplines by explaining the impact of social factors on people's experiences of health and illness. The second chapter provides further context by explaining how knowledge within the disciplines of sociology and psychology is generated through research. The next three chapters (3–5) then outline and summarise social and psychological theories relevant to pharmacy practice. One key feature of the early chapters is the use of examples to examine how theories can be interpreted for application to pharmacy practice. The very point of learning about psychosocial theories is to enable pharmacists to conduct their diverse roles in more effective ways. Pharmacists are, after all, tasked with promoting good health and better managing disease through their practice. Chapter 6 therefore bridges the gap between the psychosocial theories and their better application by examining effective modes of communication later needed for tackling the patient case studies presented in Chapter 7.

Chapter 7 tempts the reader to use the theories and methodologies outlined in the first six chapters and to relate these to pharmacy practitioners' efforts to counter-prescribe, promote good health, and to help patients with prescribed medicines through effective use of communication. The chapter is aimed at Level 1 through to Level 4 students (Year 1 of the pharmacy degree through to Masters and postgraduate levels). As recommended by the UK's Quality Assurance Agency for Higher Education, this book is written using an outcomes-based approach. Therefore throughout and in particular with the case-study chapters, the text begins by describing what a student or practitioner should know, understand and be able to demonstrate after working through the chapter. Chapter 7 contains 15 case studies (including one worked example) with questions pitched at the correct year-level, designed to meet the set learning outcomes. The idea is for readers to work through the case studies as a learning tool.

Chapter 8 focuses on research. The research case studies are aimed mainly at Level 4 students and beyond. The research cases require integration of learning from Chapter 2, which is focused on research, with theories from other chapters. A glossary is also included for important definitions.

Acknowledgements

The author would like to thank first, Louise McIndoe, Kristina Oberle and colleagues at Pharmaceutical Press for facilitating the production of this book. Thanks are also extended to colleagues in the Pharmacy Department at Reading School of Pharmacy for their efforts to ensure excellent teaching and learning practices in pharmacy. A range of pharmacy students have sampled the material in this book and the author is of course grateful for their feedback and response over the years.

Special thanks goes to various family members for facilitating time management and enabling the completion of the manuscript through their patience and understanding.

Introduction

The aim of this book is to support the teaching and learning of social and cognitive pharmacy from Level 1 of the undergraduate pharmacy course through to Level 4 and beyond. The six theory chapters focus on knowledge and understanding of a number of concepts relating to social and cognitive pharmacy, whereas the two case-study chapters aim to help learners move from mere knowledge acquisition and comprehension through to the application of knowledge, analysis, synthesis and evaluation. Thus readers working systematically through the book and to the end can be reasonably expected to meet higher-level learning outcomes necessary at Masters level and beyond.

The theory chapters should imbue the reader with not only important knowledge relating to social and cognitive pharmacy but also evidence of the usefulness of such knowledge to everyday practice. It is an undeniable fact that psychosocial factors affect beliefs and behaviour, strongly influencing people's health and illness-related outcomes. Health inequalities are especially relevant in relation to a number of significant chronic conditions such as cancer and cardiovascular diseases. The risky behaviours associated with these conditions are well established and include smoking, alcohol and drug use and obesity. Thus, pharmacists powered with relevant behavioural know-how can be reasonably expected to contribute to improving people's experience of health and illness through behavioural-change interventions.

Behaviours are linked to people's thoughts. At a basic level, thoughts and decision making have been shown to depend on people's individual preconceptions about the world and their emotional state, and this is important to understand if behaviours are to be challenged and changed. But while it is easy to assume that thoughts and therefore behaviours can be accurately and predictably mapped, research has resulted in competing models of behavioural change, none of which have been proven to be 100% effectual. Yet some of the more established and effective models present useful elements that can be applied when one is attempting to change people's behaviour from risky to more healthy practices. On a practical level, it is generally accepted that small, realisable goals, using formal contracts to specify these goals and any rewards, and monitoring and support including record-keeping, role models and positive support can potentially help the process of change. On an attitudinal level, increasing beliefs in the more negative outcomes of risky behaviour, while addressing what people perceive to be normal and also their own self-belief in their ability to change, can also help. In terms of timing, it can help to recognise people's readiness for change before attempting to embark on behaviour modification. Finally, in terms of communication, it helps to recognise people's propensity to engage differently with the information presented to them and to attempt to minimise the potential for interference and misinterpretation.

Despite preventative strategies, people find themselves facing chronic illness, and another role for the modern-day pharmacist is in supporting patients with their experience of illness and medication use, which can be especially prone to misconstrued thoughts and behaviours. Just as health behaviours depend on people's underlying attitudes and beliefs, adjustment and coping with illness too are prone to patients' inner thoughts and emotional states. People examine impending health threats in a manner that makes sense to them, judging their ability to cope as a function of available resources. Most patients' ultimate aim is to return to a state of normality. Yet, for example, when it concerns medicine taking, not all patients view pharmacological regimens in the same way as health professionals do. People's own representations of the need for medicines versus their fears about the medicines appear to be the driving factor for whether or not medicines are intentionally taken as directed, or not. Knowing this fact together with knowledge of how to change views relating to medicines can potentially help pharmacists improve and influence patients' beliefs about medicines and therefore their adherence to prescribed medication.

To implement change in practice, pharmacists must strive to use effective communication skills. Ideas relating to the ideal practitioner–patient relationship have changed over the years and nowadays health professionals are encouraged to focus on patients' needs through patient-centred care. Here, equal power-sharing, a two-way exchange of information and mutual deliberation are seen as the most effective model to adopt. Emotional intelligence too can help ease the process of communication, and becoming aware of both the impact and power of non-verbal cues can help to achieve a more successful consultation. Pharmacists can also use their knowledge of the interrelationship between thoughts and emotions to help manage their own and their patients' reactions to situations that arise in everyday practice through cognitive restructuring techniques.

Working through the patient case-study chapter engages the reader in applying these theories to a range of scenarios potentially encountered in pharmacy practice. By engaging with the cases and all accompanying tasks, readers can hone their ability to reproduce the facts and interpret the cases, indicating pertinent theories, choosing the major problems to be solved, justifying any solution, putting together their recommendation and even defending their line of reasoning through coherent argument. Working through the research case-study chapter involves readers in a different set of learning. Here, readers would have criticised any relationship between the research cases and existing theory, analysing the coherence of the research, contrasting the approach used with an opposing method, and finally questioning the underlying philosophical basis to the approach taken by the researchers in the case.

Certainly the author believes that the book has met its primary aim of being an easy-to-use medium for understanding relevant psychosocial knowledge and its application to everyday pharmacy issues. The ultimate hope of course is that such learning equips the next generation of pharmacists with the confidence needed for even greater impact on population health and patient care.

Parastou Donyai
London, UK

1

Importance of sociology and psychology to pharmacy practice

Synopsis

This chapter outlines the importance of sociology and psychology to the practice of pharmacy. First it provides an overview of the subjects of sociology and psychology as they relate to pharmacy, then it examines the interrelationship between social factors and people's experiences of health and illness. In doing so, it provides the framework for the book's main rationale, that to be more effective, pharmacists need to be aware of the breadth of factors affecting health. This is so that pharmacists can, in turn, use their knowledge of social and cognitive pharmacy to impact on people's beliefs and behaviour at an individual level via everyday practice.

Learning outcomes

After working through this chapter, you should be able to demonstrate knowledge and understanding of:

- the need to study social and cognitive pharmacy
- the relationship between social factors and health and illness.

Introduction

Humans live in communities and interact with each other in countless ways. People's lives are social and involve relations to others. A collection of people sharing common traditions, institutions, territories, activities and interests is known as a society. In simple terms, a society is thought of as something that exists beyond the individual subject; for example, one speaks of British society. This common-sense usage of the term is particularly helpful for beginners. Sociology is the scientific study of society, including the study of the development, structure and functioning of human society, and patterns of social relationships, social action and culture. Sociologists are concerned with providing descriptions of social phenomena and trends and analysing prevailing social problems. Contemporary sociology is subdivided into many specific fields within which sociologists can take one of a number of philosophical standpoints. Selecting from a range of associated research methodology, sociologists generate or test new hypotheses, leading to the enrichment of the discipline in an iterative process. Modern sociology has an interface with public health in a number of ways, including medical sociology, which involves the use of sociological knowledge to aid diagnosis, treatment, teaching and research in medicine. In recent years, interest in the application of sociology to pharmacy practice has led to the development of a new discipline. Pharmaceutical sociology (sometimes referred to as *social pharmacy*) is concerned with the social institution of pharmacy and society as it relates to patients, medicines and the work of the pharmacist.

Exploring the concept: sociology

Another way to think about sociology and how it relates to pharmacy is to think of it as a way of helping us understand, for example, why pharmacists seem to behave in predictable ways at work or why the public seem to be influenced in their health behaviour by the social group they are in. Let's take the first example further by thinking about a practice such as independent prescribing. Whether a pharmacist becomes an independent prescriber is no doubt influenced by their individual choices and preferences. The pharmacist, for example, may have wanted to study further to gain independent-prescriber status. However, further reflection and research will in fact reveal that independent prescribing is also strongly influenced by factors that are social in origin. First, regulations to allow independent prescribing by pharmacists only came into effect in May 2006. Before that, the concept of independent prescribing was not a reality. Second, research has shown that pharmacists with independent-prescribing qualifications do not necessarily go on to practise it. For example, reactions from medical colleagues as well as local policy makers can make it difficult for pharmacists to practise independent prescribing in some instances. This suggests then that pharmacists' practice is subject to change and is also something that is shared and shaped by social factors. Social pharmacy tries to investigate and provide a sense of understanding about such phenomena.

While sociology is concerned with studying groups of people, psychology involves studying people at the level of the individual. Psychologists are interested essentially in what makes us human. Psychology is the study of the human mind and its functions as it relates to human behaviour, cognition (thought) and experience. Psychology is also a diverse, multi-perspective discipline with roots in medicine, philosophy, biology as well as physiology. Many concepts classified as psychological also have practical implication for how people live in communities and interact with each other. Psychology influences society in many ways and distinct elements of psychology are concerned with the application of research findings to solving human problems at societal level. Social psychology is concerned with studying the psychology of social interactions. For example, psychologists can examine the mental processing of social knowledge through what is known as social cognition.

Psychology can also be related to health and illness and the work of health professionals. For example, medical psychology is concerned with problems that arise in medicine including psychological aspects of pain, terminal illness, bereavement, disability and reactions to medical advice, whereas health psychology is concerned with psychological aspect of health promotion, disease prevention, treatment and identification of psychological causes and patterns of health and illness. A more recent addition is occupational health psychology, which is concerned with the application of psychology to improving the quality of people's work and the protection and promotion of the health, safety and well-being of those at work. Here, the term pharmaceutical psychology can be coined to describe the study of people's beliefs and behaviour in relation to the activities of the modern-day pharmacist, from experiences with health promotion and disease diagnosis in the pharmacy to beliefs and behaviours relating to the prescribing, counter-prescribing, review and dispensing of the full range of pharmacologically active compounds by pharmacists. In this context, cognitive pharmacy involves pharmacy-relevant thoughts and beliefs, with the term *cognitive pharmacy services* being used specifically to denote structured attempts to change patients' behaviour through the practice of pharmacy.

Exploring the concept: psychology

Another way to think about psychology and how it relates to pharmacy is to think of it as a way of helping us understand, for example, why some patients are likely to adhere to their medication regimen, while others are not. Research has shown that around half of all patients on chronic medication do not take these as intended by the prescriber. One theorist, Horne (see Chapter 5), claims that patients' adherence to medication can be predicted by the balance of their concerns about the medicines versus the necessity of taking them. Horne's necessity–concerns framework deals directly with the patient's internal thought processes in relation to the medicine; in other words, the psychology of the medication. Other psychological theories relating to pharmacy are examined in later chapters.

This book in fact deals with the impact of both sociology and psychology on pharmacy practice and is concerned specifically with social and cognitive pharmacy.

Studying social and cognitive pharmacy

To further understand the relevance of psychosocial theories to pharmacy practice, let us start by examining the limitation of 'biology' in explaining all health outcomes. Picture the human brain. It contains more than 100 billion neurons, specialised cells that convey and process information using electrical signals and the release of chemicals. Biochemical analyses have shown that chemical neurotransmitters exist within neurons and are released from one neuron to communicate with the next after crossing the synaptic gap (between the neurons). Biology teaches us that the activity of neural systems can alter information processing in the brain and in turn affect thought, mood and behaviour. For example, a decrease in levels of the neurotransmitter serotonin is associated with depression while an increase in synaptic serotonin levels, achieved by blocking the reuptake of serotonin into the neuron, say with a drug, can reverse some of the signs of depression. But is all behaviour driven solely through biological changes? And which comes first – does a reduction in serotonin levels result in depression, or do depressing thoughts lower serotonin levels? Although studying the brain has helped provide an understanding of the relationship between brain activity (biology) and behaviour (human action) this relationship is far from straightforward. A reductionist approach would trim down behaviour to biology only. However, it is now accepted that psychosocial factors impact on behaviour to a greater extent than biology alone, strongly influencing people's health and illness-related outcomes.

Exploring the concept: reductionism

Drugs that inhibit the reuptake of serotonin can be, and indeed are, used as antidepressants. Serotonergic neurons are involved in thought and mood, therefore increasing the presence of serotonin at the synapses can alter information processing in the brain to result in mood elevation. Indeed, in addition to mechanistic studies, clinical trials (planned human experiments) have demonstrated a positive correlation between administering selective serotonin reuptake inhibitors (SSRIs) to patients and mood elevation, and for this reason SSRIs are licensed as antidepressant drugs in the United Kingdom. The effect of pharmacological intervention in humans, however, must be taken in the context of the person as a whole. For example, the drug paroxetine, an SSRI, can also increase suicidal thoughts and rates of suicide in certain patient groups. This is opposite to what is expected if that expectation is based purely on the pharmacology of the drug. Indeed, paroxetine should not be used in the treatment of children and adolescents under the age of 18 years because it can induce suicidal ideation in this group. Although paroxetine is an antidepressant, in this example the outcome observed in clinical practice is different to the expected pharmacological effect. This is because the link between brain activity and behaviour is far from straightforward. Analysis of outcomes purely on a biological level will miss other determining factors such as the psychological and social context. Likewise, a non-pharmacological treatment for depression involving cognitive behaviour therapy is now understood to be effective in lowering depression by consciously altering thought processes that impact on the brain, without the aid of drugs, to result in the enhancement of mood. In this way, thought (cognition) and behaviour affect brain activity and mood, rather than vice versa. A purely biological perspective using reductionism could not provide sufficient explanation of the phenomena.

In reality, not all behaviour can be fully and simplistically accounted for in terms of biological (or biomedical) explanations and so modern-day psychologists use their understanding of biology to bolster their theories on human action rather than solely to explain them. Similarly, one could argue that it would be too simplistic to expect the modern-day pharmacist to be solely concerned with a pharmacological intervention without taking into account the patient's social and psychological context, which can influence their health-related behaviour to a great extent. What an individual thinks and how they behave within a socioeconomic framework can have a substantial effect on their health, experience of illness and disease management.

Pharmacists nowadays are tasked with promoting good health, diagnosing disease, prescribing medicines and ensuring adherence. Although the natural sciences of pharmacy provide essential underpinning knowledge, it can no longer suffice to depend solely on knowledge of pharmaceutical chemistry, pharmacology and pharmaceutics to be an effective pharmacist. The involvement of pharmacists in a range of extended roles and activities now necessitates an in-depth understanding and application of the behavioural sciences. For example, there is evidence that the application of psychological theories can help pharmacists influence patients' beliefs about health and illness and therefore behaviour such as adherence to medication. Social and cognitive pharmacy is concerned with the application of psychosocial knowledge to impact on patients' health and illness-related behaviour within the context of practice.

But before examining health-related social and psychological theories and their application to pharmacy, an acknowledgement of the bio-psychosocial model of health is necessary. In fact, a common way of relating sociology and psychology to health is to explain initially the biomedical model of health and its limitations, before highlighting the more complete nature of the bio-psychosocial model and therefore its greater usefulness for understanding people's actual experiences of health and illness. Here, the distinction between the biomedical and the bio-psychosocial models is elucidated in the context of the more detailed philosophical discussions in Chapter 2, which explain that epistemology – theories about 'how we know what we know' – defines what should count as knowledge when conducting research. In the same vein, epistemology can also define what should count as knowledge in operational terms, for example, in relation to views about health and illness. Which view should define one's understanding of health – can a biomedical explanation of disease suffice?

For a number of centuries, based on the philosophical ideas of Francis Bacon (1561–1626), and René Descartes (1596–1650), the practice of medicine in the West has followed the biomedical model of health and disease as underpinned by the empiricist tradition. To understand this better, you are invited to examine in detail the assumptions of empiricism and positivism outlined in Chapter 2. The ultimate idea of the biomedical model, in line with the assumptions of positivism, is that the whole can be considered as the sum of its parts and that therefore medical problems can be addressed at the population, individual, organ, tissue, cellular and molecular levels. Of course, no one would dispute the contribution of science and medicine to the progress of humankind. However, critics of the biomedical model would argue that it encourages a reductionist approach that fails to account for problems when the whole is *different* from the sum of its parts.

Thus, there arises an ontological dilemma. While the concept of ontology is further examined in Chapter 2, for now let's consider this dilemma: what does it mean to be human?

The interpretative approach, explained further in Chapter 2, makes a case for human complexity, where people's interactions and subjectivity matter just as much as, if not more than, their biomedical particulars. To be human is to be embodied and to live among other people, and interact with them and be influenced by them in countless ways. Thus as an alternative to the biomedical model, the bio-psychosocial model acknowledges a complex interaction of biological, psychological and social factors in influencing health and disease. This could even include the influence of pharmacy on patients' health. The main aim of this book is to help students of pharmacy and pharmacists understand and use relevant psychosocial theories in their work and everyday practice.

Relevance of sociology to pharmacy

One could argue that not too many individuals (let alone pharmacists – but of course that is not meant as a criticism) can exert influence at a policy level, and therefore have an effect on the wider society. However, appreciating social influences on people's experiences of health and illness at least provides sufficient justification for why pharmacists are being called to help change people's behaviour at the individual level, through suitable services and interventions. Thus the focus of the remainder of this chapter is to introduce some of the findings that sociology offers pharmacy, as a basis for the ensuing chapters that focus on behaviour change. This is because what pharmacists *are* potentially able to influence, with the right training and on a one-to-one basis, is the behaviour of the patient. Therefore, the main aim of the remainder of the theory chapters is to provide relevant psychological know-how to equip pharmacists with the tools required to affect their patients' health and illness-related behaviour at the individual level. However, as explained above, for now some broader concepts are examined that help explain why patients may behave in the way that they do because of wider influences.

It was stated above that sociology is the scientific study of the development, structure and functioning of human society, and patterns of social relationships, social action and culture, and that sociologists are concerned with providing descriptions of social phenomena and trends and analysing prevailing social problems. What can sociology tell us about patients? For one, it is an undisputed fact that social factors influence people's health, be it in a health-promoting or a health-damaging way. Thus, in the first instance, sociology can help pharmacists gain a better understanding of why people experience health differently according to their social, economic or political situations.

Social determinants of health

The impact of absolute material deprivation (such as inadequate food, clothing, shelter, water and sanitation) on health has been recognised for centuries. However, nowadays it is also recognised that people's health is not only shaped by material deprivation and their living and working conditions but also by economic and social resources, and even by opportunities that influence their access to health-promoting behaviours and healthy choices. According to the World Health Organization (WHO) the social determinants of health are 'the conditions in which people are born, grow, live, work and age, including the health system'. In addition, WHO recognises that the social determinants of health in themselves 'are shaped by the distribution of money, power and resources at global, national and local levels, which are themselves influenced by policy choices'. This broader definition attempts to capture the many complex factors that can affect people's experiences of health and illness. The main message is that social determinants of health are responsible for health inequities – the unfair and avoidable differences in health status seen within and between countries.

As introduced above, the social determinants of health concern the structural determinants and conditions of daily life, more specifically the distribution of power, income, goods and services, globally and nationally, as well as the immediate, visible circumstances of people's lives, such as their access to healthcare, schools and education, their conditions of work and leisure, their homes, communities, and rural or urban settings and their chances of leading a flourishing life. In 2008, the WHO Commission on Social Determinants of Health, which was established to support countries to address the social factors leading to ill health and inequities, produced a report entitled *Closing the Gap in a Generation: Health equity through action on the social determinants of health*. Its overarching recommendations were:

- to improve daily conditions
- to tackle the inequitable distribution of money, power and resources
- to measure and understand.

The WHO report is helpful in focusing attention on the social determinants of health across the world, and the far-reaching recommendations serve to provide a basis for action by governments and policymakers. Yet, people in the developed countries encounter a subset of the global social influences on health, which are worth examining in their own right.

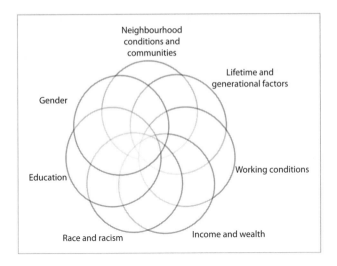

Figure 1.1 Some of the social determinants of health. (Data from Braveman *et al.* 2011.)

In England, the 'Marmot Review' published in 2010 was a comprehensive study of health inequalities in England (Marmot *et al.* 2010). It too resulted in recommendations that, in fact, later made up the body of a 2010 UK government policy paper on tackling health inequalities. Of course, health inequalities have persisted over time and before the review by Marmot; among others there were the reports by Black (Department of Health and Social Security 1980) and Acheson (1998) in the UK. This section draws on the Marmot Review and a comprehensive review of the published literature on the social determinants of health in the developed countries by Braveman *et al.* published in 2011. They examined the influence of several social factors on people's health, including neighbourhood conditions, working conditions, education, income and wealth, race and racism, and the all-encompassing factor of stress. The findings of these papers are drawn upon to outline below the social determinants of health in the developed world, as a basis for the discussions (Figure 1.1).

Neighbourhood conditions, communities and health

According Braveman *et al.* (2011), people's neighbourhoods can affect their health through physical factors such as water and air quality and closeness to hazardous substances; housing-related factors such as overcrowding and exposure to pest infestation, lead paint, mould and dust; and other factors such as access to food and an environment for exercise, green spaces, air quality, fuel poverty as well as safety from traffic. Additional factors can also play a role, for example, the quality of local services such as schools, transportation, medical care and employment resources as well as social relations.

Here, mutual trust and understanding within a neighbourhood are thought to be linked to lower levels of crime with the converse situation leading to more disorder and depression and anxiety among residents. According to the Marmot Review too the physical and social characteristics of communities and the degree to which they enable healthy behaviours all impact on health inequalities (Marmot *et al.* 2010).

Other factors considered in the Marmot Review are those relating to sustainable communities and the effects of climate change (Marmot *et al.* 2010). Although this may appear to be a futuristic concern, at the time of writing this book, in Japan the earthquake and catastrophic tsunami that ensued, together with the threat of radiation leaking from the earthquake-damaged nuclear reactor all serve as stark reminders that the weather, be it extreme temperatures, natural disasters or the effects of ozone depletion, can all affect health and indeed life itself at any point. People on low incomes are thought less likely to be able to afford protection against adversities brought about by climate change. As well as a direct impact, climate change is also affecting the price and availability of food and this effect too will be most felt by the more deprived communities.

Working conditions and health

People's working conditions can impact on health in the following ways according to the evidence presented in the review by Braveman *et al.* (2011). The simplest consideration is the physical nature of people's work. For example, jobs requiring high physical workload or repetitive movements put the employees at higher risk of injuries and musculoskeletal disorders. Conversely, jobs that result in physical inactivity increase employees' risk of diabetes, heart disease and obesity. Other occupational factors affecting health include unsatisfactory ventilation, noise levels and exposure to hazardous chemicals. As well as physical factors, dangerous work, lack of safety, long working hours, shift-work and irregular working hours can also impact on health. Psychosocial aspects of work are thought to influence health, with working overtime, for example, thought to be a factor in injury, illness and death.

Similarly, jobs placing employees under high duress, especially where the employee has little control or where there is a perceived lack of meritocracy are also thought to result in risks of poorer health. Other work-based influences on health are thought to include control at work generally, social support, and of course work-related opportunities and resources such as earnings and benefits, which can affect living conditions. Employees can feel they have little control at work – for example, when there are conflicts within hierarchies or when they are restricted in decision-making processes or there are discriminatory practices in place. According to the Marmot

Review a toxic combination of work-related factors can occur among the most deprived workers, especially with precarious jobs that can involve low wages and job instability (Marmot *et al.* 2010). A range of conditions are associated with the psychosocial hazards of work and the resulting stress including mental illness, cardiovascular diseases and diabetes.

In addition, according to the Marmot Review, although being in *good* employment is protective of health, being unemployed also contributes to poor health (Marmot *et al.* 2010). Patterns of employment though can reflect existing social disparities, for example, in terms of access to the labour market, with unemployment rates being higher for those with no or fewer qualifications and skills, the mentally ill, people with disabilities, single parents, those from ethnic minorities, older workers and even young people. Even when these groups do gain employment, it seems they are more likely to have poor-quality jobs with lower pay and opportunities for advancement, experiencing more harmful health effects. According to the Marmot Review, unemployment can exert its effect on health via financial consequences, distress and anxiety and unhealthy behaviours such as alcohol abuse and lack of exercise, and is associated with limiting long-term illness, mental illness and cardiovascular disease, higher medication use, as well as overall mortality and suicide.

Education and health

Another main factor concerning health, according to the evidence, is the educational level of the individual. For example, education can increase literacy, including health literacy, affecting choices and healthy behaviours. Education can also influence employment opportunities, impacting on health via economic resources, with more educated individuals experiencing lower rates of unemployment, which as described above is associated with illness and higher mortality rates. More educated individuals are also thought to benefit from healthier work conditions (physical and psychosocial) as well as, of course, higher pay and employment-related benefits. Higher educational achievement is also thought to impinge on people's perception of control, social standing, and social support resulting in better health and healthier behaviours via a number of different routes.

Income, wealth and health

Access to economic resources can affect people's health. While wealth, which describes accumulated material assets such as a home and vehicles, may better reflect economic resources overall, it is income (i.e., earnings over a defined time period) that has been used in studies of health because it is easier to measure. However, Braveman *et al.* (2011) explain that studies that have examined wealth (after accounting for income) do also find a link with health. Some have argued that reverse causation may explain the relationship between income and health (with poor health resulting in income loss) but this is not generally thought to account for the association between income and health. The ultimate finding is that increasing income is associated with better health, and this may well be via other socioeconomic factors such as educational achievement and quality, childhood circumstances, impact of the neighbourhood, working conditions and perceived social status. The relationship between low income and poor health could also be explained by people's inability to purchase goods and services that maintain or improve their health. Being poor can also stop people participating in social events resulting in a lower sense of esteem and societal worth.

In addition, income inequality at a societal level is often linked with health – thus nations with a smaller difference between the rich and the poor are shown to have better overall health. This may reflect other factors such as lack of social cohesion and social solidarity, which could be a cause or effect of income inequality. An often talked-about book by Wilkinson and Pickett (2010) called *The Spirit Level* describes the relationship between inequality and health outcomes and could be read for further awareness.

Race, racism and health

Another important determinant of health in Western countries is race or ethnic origin, for example, through racism. Braveman *et al.* (2011) explain that racism need not refer to overt, intentional discrimination but inherent structures and societal systems that inadvertently discriminate and affect some individuals' life chances and resources based on their ethnic background. A typical example is living in an area in accordance with one's race, resulting in neighbourhoods that are inadequately resourced in turn, for example, leading to lower educational achievement for the residents with the ensuing impact on health as discussed above. Racism could also influence health through long-term stress on the individual resulting from others' ethnic bias or even the accumulation of subtle, everyday experiences that transcend the individual's neighbourhood, income or educational attainment.

Impact of stress

One way in which the social factors outlined above could influence health is via the mediating effect of stress. Dealing with life's challenges in less desirable social circumstances can be stressful and evidence links some of the social determinants with poorer health through the impact of chronic stress on the neuroendocrine system, inflammatory pathways, immune mechanism and/or vascular effects. This is because stressful events and experiences, as well as psychosocial causes (e.g., perceived control and social status) can all trigger the release of cytokines, cortisol and other mediators that adversely affect vital organs and the body's immune defences, over time leading to the progression or more rapid development of chronic diseases such as cardiovascular disease. Stress can also lead to the uptake of risky health behaviours as a method of coping. The topic of stress and its effect on health is itself the subject of a chapter if not a separate book. For further information, see excellent reviews by Miller *et al.* (2009), Umberson *et al.* (2010) and Matthews and Gallo (2011).

Other groups in society

According to the Marmot Review, as well as the factors examined above, a number of other domains are associated with social inequalities including age, gender, religion, language and mental health and sexual orientation. In addition, in the UK there are the homeless, and refugees and asylum seekers, including people who receive little or no financial support which can ensure they remain in absolute poverty. These differences interact with people's socioeconomic position to affect their health. For example, people with learning or physical disabilities may suffer more discrimination, have poorer access to health services and less desirable employment, all of which have an impact on their health status. Of course, it is too simple to assume that health outcomes can be associated with one factor only – in reality it is the multi-factorial nature of socioeconomic disadvantage that produces health inequalities.

Lifetime and generational factors

In addition to factors encountered through the course of life, early experiences in childhood (especially in the first five years of life) in families facing social disadvantage, can also have an adverse effect on health. Childhood experiences lay down a basis for the whole of one's life. This is because early experiences (e.g., lack of stimulation from parents/carers) can shape children's mental, behavioural and physical development, in turn later affecting health, for example, through readiness for school, educational attainment and economic participation. Thus childhood experiences can influence health and disadvantage throughout life.

Even before birth, the health and well-being of the mother during pregnancy can impact on the development of the foetus through such behaviours as maternal depression, stress, obesity, alcohol abuse and smoking. Some of these can affect the birthweight of the baby and certainly low birthweight is associated with poorer long-term health and educational outcomes for the child. In-utero factors are also thought to have an effect on the foetus's brain development and even the risk of cardiovascular diseases in later life.

Certainly, low birthweight is associated with the mother's socioeconomic circumstances. According to the Marmot Review, children from disadvantaged backgrounds are more likely to begin school with lower personal, social and emotional development and communication, language and literacy skills than their peers.

In addition, research has shown there are more overarching intergenerational effects. For example, children of socially disadvantaged parents do not learn about educational opportunities resulting in social disadvantage for them later in adulthood. In addition, poor parent–child relationships could weaken children's self-esteem and confidence and in turn increase their risk of adopting unhealthy lifestyles as adults. Other developmental factors that can affect later health include childhood obesity, which in some Western countries is becoming the norm. In addition, risky adolescent behaviours such as cannabis use, smoking, sexual experimentation and drunkenness can also influence health.

One last life-course determinant of health to consider is ageing itself. People in the West have higher life expectancies than ever before, yet can suffer from loneliness and in turn depression, through deteriorating social ties and family networks. Older people may also have dementia, which may be vascular in origin and therefore linked to diet and lifestyle.

Gender differences

An additional factor often related to differences in health outcomes is that of gender. It is a well-accepted fact that women, on average, live longer than men and various explanations account for this difference. A variety of biological explanations have been proposed for the observed higher rates of mortality in men, which include the beneficial effects of female sex hormones on the cardiovascular system, and the risk-inducing effect of testosterone in men resulting in higher accident rates and therefore death. There is also the hypothesis that genes present in the additional X chromosome in females compensate for genes on the first X chromosome which may have been damaged – with age for example.

On the other hand, non-biological theories focus on sociocultural influences and behavioural factors in explaining the higher mortality rates found in men. For example, traditionally it is thought that men are more likely to engage in risky employment such as heavy manufacturing, to take up unhealthy behaviours such as smoking and drinking and to have unhealthy diets and make less use of health services for disease prevention and treatment. It could also be that men suffer greater levels of social stress as a result of their social standing and professional lives. For example, the spring 2011 issue of the British Office for National Statistics publication, *Health Statistics Quarterly*, reported a one-year increase in the life expectancy gap between men in the most and least advantaged social groups, despite an overall improvement for all groups. In reality, it could be a combination of both biological and sociobehavioural factors that account for the higher mortality rates in men. The next section provides a summary of health outcomes data for England and Wales, valid as of spring 2011.

Health outcomes data

It was argued above that health is determined by a complex interaction of social, economic and political circumstances. But what is in fact meant by health? Health is defined in the WHO constitution of 1948 as: 'A state of complete physical, social and mental well-being, and not merely the absence of disease or infirmity'.

Within the context of health promotion, health has been expressed in functional terms 'as a resource which permits people to lead an individually, socially and economically productive life'. The WHO Ottawa Charter for Health Promotion (1986) considers health as a resource for everyday life, not the object of living; as such health 'is a positive concept emphasising social and personal resources as well as physical capabilities'. Health is regarded by WHO as a fundamental human right, and correspondingly, all people should have access to basic resources for health. In keeping with the concept of health as a fundamental human right, the Ottawa Charter emphasises certain prerequisites for health which include 'peace, adequate economic resources, food and shelter, and a stable eco-system and sustainable resource use'. This way of thinking emphasises the links between social and economic conditions, the physical environment, individual lifestyles and health.

To provide a clearer picture of the link between social circumstances and health, it is worth examining in more detail some of the evidence of the health inequalities referred to in the section above. In England and Wales, the Office for National Statistics (ONS) is a government body responsible for collecting and analysing population-level data, which includes the collection of health-related data. One of the measures used by the ONS to examine health statistics across society is the socioeconomic classification. The National Statistics Socio-economic Classification (NS-SEC) was introduced in 2001 (and updated in 2005) to replace previous classifications including the Registrar General's Social Class (SC) and Socio-economic Group (SEG). NS-SEC is based on occupation but has the capacity to cover the adult population including, for example, the long-term unemployed and students (Table 1.1).

Other ways in which health statistics are expressed include stratification according to gender, geographical region and ethnicity. In light of the discussions above that highlight a complex relationship between social determinants of health, it is interesting to note that there are marked differences

Table 1.1 The eight-class grouping of the National Statistics Socio-economic Classification (NS-SEC) used by the Office for National Statistics for its analyses. (Data from ONS 2005.)

Classification title	Description	Example occupations
1. Higher managerial and professional occupations	Includes employers in large organisations, managerial professions and higher professional occupations	Chief executives of major organisations, doctors, lawyers, architects, professors
2. Lower managerial and professional occupations	Includes lower professional and higher technical occupations, lower managerial occupations and higher supervisory occupations	School teachers, social workers, actors, nurses, journalists, police sergeants
3. Intermediate occupations	Positions in clerical, sales and intermediate technical occupations that do not involve general planning or supervisory powers	Civil Service administrative officers, secretaries, firemen, auxiliary nurses, photographers, airline cabin crew
4. Small employers and own-account workers	Those who employ others on a small scale. Own-account workers are self-employed and have no employees other than family	Shopkeepers, farmers, non-professionals with fewer than 25 employees such as builders and hairdressers
5. Lower supervisory and technical occupations	Lower supervisory occupations have titles such as 'foreman' and 'supervisor' and have formal and immediate supervision over those in classes 6 and 7	Plumbers, motor mechanics, electricians, taxi drivers
6. Semi-routine occupations	Work requires at least some element of employee discretion/decision making	Traffic wardens, farm workers, shop assistants, postmen, security guards
7. Routine occupations	Positions with a basic labour contract, where employees are paid for the specific service; less employee discretion/decision making required	Bus drivers, cleaners, waitresses, refuse collectors, car park attendants
8. Never-worked and long-term unemployed	Have never had an occupation or have been unemployed for an extended period and can therefore not be assigned to an NS-SEC category. 'Long-term' can be defined as any period of time but is generally one or two years	
Not classified (including full-time students, occupations not stated or inadequately described and not classifiable for other reasons)	There is insufficient information to classify the individual. Other reasons include, e.g., retirement, long-term illness and disability, people looking after the home and short-term unemployed when a previous occupation cannot be found. Full-time students normally recorded as students, even if a previous occupation is given	

in NS-SEC across gender, geographical region as well as ethnicity. For example, overall, men are more than twice as likely as women to be in higher managerial and professional occupations (15.2% vs 6.9%, respectively),

Table 1.2 National Statistics Socio-economic Classification and gender for working-age men (16–64 years) and women (16–59 years) based on the 'labour force survey' conducted in autumn 2005 for the Office for National Statistics. (Data from Hall 2006.)

NS-SEC analytical class	Men (%)	Women (%)
1. Higher managerial and professional occupations	15.2	6.9
2. Lower managerial and professional occupations	20.4	24.6
3. Intermediate occupations	5.2	15.0
4. Small employers and own-account workers	11.1	4.1
5. Lower supervisory and technical occupations	12.6	5.4
6. Semi-routine occupations	9.5	16.3
7. Routine occupations	11.3	7.3
8. Never-worked and long-term unemployed	3.2	4.4
Full-time students and unclassified	11.5	16.0
Total	100	100

whereas intermediate occupations consistently have a greater representation of women than men (15.0% vs 5.2%, respectively) (Table 1.2). Men are more likely than women to be in lower supervisory and technical occupations (12.6% vs 5.4%, respectively), whereas those in semi-routine occupations are more likely to be women than men (16.3% vs 9.5%). In terms of geographical region, according to Ashton and Kent (2008), reviewing data from the annual population survey for the ONS in 2004, the highest representation of people in higher managerial and professional occupations is in the southern regions of the UK, particularly around London, with much lower concentrations further north. The contrasting pattern is shown by the proportions in routine and manual occupations with the greatest concentrations being found in the north of England, Wales and Scotland.

In terms of ethnicity and NS-SEC, according to Dobbs *et al.* (2006) reporting on the Census 2001 data, Bangladeshi and Pakistani men in employment have the lowest proportion working in 'managerial and professional occupations' (23% and 29% for Bangladeshi and Pakistani, respectively), and the highest proportion working in 'semi-routine and routine occupations' (43% and 34%, respectively). In contrast, black African, Indian, white British, and Chinese men had a higher proportion working in 'managerial and professional occupations' (47%, 46%, 42%, and 44%, respectively) and a lower proportion in 'semi-routine and routine occupations' (25%, 23%, 24%, and 19%, respectively). The pattern was similar for women in employment in 2001, with Bangladeshi and Pakistani women again having the lowest proportion working in 'managerial and professional occupations' (32% and 34%, respectively) and the highest working in 'semi-routine and routine occupations' (35% and 33%, respectively). In comparison with men, white British and Indian women in employment had a lower proportion working in 'managerial and professional occupations' (38%, and 37%, respectively) and a higher proportion working in 'semi-routine and routine occupations' (29% and 30%, respectively). Interestingly, black African, black Caribbean and Chinese women reported a higher proportion working in 'managerial and professional occupations' (44%, 44%, and 43%) compared with their Indian and white British counterparts.

Returning to health inequalities, whether stratified according to socio-economic class, gender, geographical region or ethnicity, inequity can be expressed and demonstrated using a number of health outcomes, including life expectancy, mortality figures, morbidity figures, self-reported health, mental health, death and injury from accidents and violence. Here, the focus is first on examining patterns of life expectancy, mortality rates and self-reported health before considering patterns of health behaviours associated with mortality and disease.

Life expectancy in the UK

The latest figures on male and female life expectancy at birth for local areas in the UK that were available in the spring of 2011 related to 2007–2009 (ONS 2010a). One of the key messages from these statistics is that, as per previous findings, inequalities exist and persist across the UK. The southeast, southwest and east of England have the highest life expectancies at birth, whereas these figures are lowest in Scotland and in the northwest and northeast of England. Despite this, it is worth noting that life expectancy in general is increasing in the UK (Figure 1.2).

In terms of inequalities, however, the 2007–2009 statistics (ONS 2010a) showed firstly that life expectancy *at birth* for males was highest in the southeast of England (79.4 years) and lowest in Scotland (75.4 years), representing a difference of 4.0 years between the two regions. As alluded to above, women live longer than men in the Western world; so the highest life expectancy at birth for females was 83.3 years (in the southeast and southwest of England) and the lowest was 80.1 years (in Scotland), representing a 3.2 years difference between the two regions. Similarly, life expectancy *at age 65* was highest for males in the southeast of England (a further 18.7 years to live) and highest for females in the southeast and southwest of England (a further 21.3 years to live). Again, Scotland had the lowest life expectancy at age 65 for both males and females with a further 16.5 years and 19.1 years to live, respectively.

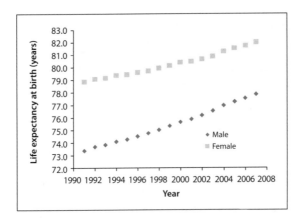

Figure 1.2 Life expectancy at birth in the UK for males and females 1991–1993 to 2007–2009. (Data from ONS 2010a.)

When the figures were published, a much-talked-about difference in life expectancy related to people living in the affluent London borough of Kensington and Chelsea (84.4 years for males and 89.0 years for females at birth and a further 23.7 years for males and 26.5 years for females, at age 65) compared with that of people living in the deprived area of Glasgow city (71.1 years for males and 77.5 years for females, at birth and a further 13.9 years for males and 17.6 years for females at age 65). This meant that men born in Glasgow could on average expect to live 13.3 fewer years than men born in Kensington and Chelsea, with women expecting to live 11.5 fewer years. Certainly, there is a gradient of decreasing life expectancy at birth and at age 65 in moving down the social scale for both men and women for the past three decades (Table 1.3).

Mortality figures in England and Wales

The latest figures on male and female deaths registered in England and Wales that were available in the spring of 2011 related to 2009 (ONS 2010b). A total of 491 348 deaths were registered in England and Wales in 2009 (compared with 509 090 in 2008). This translated to an age-standardised mortality rate of 6573 deaths per million population for males and 4628 deaths per million for females. In terms of the infant mortality rate (deaths under one year of age), this was 4.7 deaths per 1000 live births in 2009 (compared with 4.8 in 2008). Again, it is worth contextualising that, according to the ONS, the infant mortality rate in 2009 (based on registrations) was the lowest ever recorded in England and Wales.

Looking at causes of death, the highest age-standardised mortality rate in 2009 was for circulatory diseases, with 2078 deaths per million population for men and 1312 deaths per million population for women. The largest

Table 1.3 The trend in life expectancy for men and women at birth according to National Statistics Socio-economic Classification. (Data from ONS 2010a.)

NS-SEC analytical class	Life expectancy at birth (years)				
	1982–86	1987–91	1992–96	1997–2001	2002–2006
Men					
1. Higher managerial and professional	75.6	76.6	77.5	78.8	80.4
2. Lower managerial and professional occupations	74.3	75.4	76.5	78.2	79.6
3. Intermediate occupations	73.3	74.5	75.3	76.8	78.5
4. Small employers and own-account workers	73.6	74.4	75.6	76.6	77.8
5. Lower supervisory and technical occupations	72.3	73.2	73.8	75.3	76.8
6. Semi-routine occupations	71.3	71.7	72.4	74.0	75.1
7. Routine occupations	70.7	71.5	71.6	72.6	74.6
Women					
1. Higher managerial and professional	80.9	81.7	82.3	82.6	83.9
2. Lower managerial and professional occupations	79.7	81.0	81.2	82.2	83.4
3. Intermediate occupations	79.6	81.1	81.4	81.5	82.7
4. Small employers and own-account workers	79.1	79.9	80.7	80.8	82.6
5. Lower supervisory and technical occupations	78.5	78.1	79.4	79.5	80.4
6. Semi-routine occupations	78.1	78.5	79.2	79.6	80.6
7. Routine occupations	77.1	77.5	78.3	78.6	79.7

overall number of deaths in England and Wales in 2009 related to circulatory diseases, which include ischaemic heart diseases and strokes (33% of all deaths), cancers (29% of all deaths), and respiratory diseases, which include deaths from pneumonia (14% of all deaths). For both men and women, the leading cause of death is ischaemic heart diseases, accounting for about a sixth of deaths in men and an eighth of deaths in women in England and Wales in 2009 (Table 1.4). The second leading cause of death in men is lung cancer, accounting for over 7% of all male deaths in 2009, while in women this is cerebrovascular diseases (strokes), accounting for over 10% of female deaths in 2009. For both men and women, lung cancer was the most common cancer recorded as cause of death.

Table 1.4 Leading causes of mortality by gender in England and Wales, 2009. (Data from ONS 2010b.)

Ranked by number of deaths	Underlying cause of death	Number of deaths	Percentage of all deaths	Age-standardised, all-age mortality rate per 100 000 population
Males				
1	Ischaemic heart diseases	41 455	17.4	113.0
2	Malignant neoplasm of trachea, bronchus and lung	17 053	7.2	48.0
3	Cerebrovascular diseases	16 888	7.1	43.2
4	Chronic lower respiratory diseases	13 165	5.5	34.2
5	Influenza and pneumonia	11 108	4.7	28.4
6	Malignant neoplasm of prostate	9402	3.9	23.9
7	Malignant neoplasm of colon, sigmoid, rectum and anus	7559	3.2	21.0
8	Dementia and Alzheimer's disease	6709	2.8	16.2
9	Malignant neoplasms of lymphoid, haematopoietic and related tissue	5922	2.5	16.6
10	Diseases of the liver	4604	1.9	15.7
	All male deaths	238 062		
Females				
1	Ischaemic heart diseases	30 725	12.1	50.4
2	Cerebrovascular diseases	26 707	10.5	40.7
3	Dementia and Alzheimer's disease	15 909	6.3	21.5
4	Influenza and Pneumonia	15 711	6.2	22.9
5	Malignant neoplasm of trachea, bronchus and lung	12 965	5.1	29.8
6	Chronic lower respiratory diseases	12 254	4.8	23.0
7	Neoplasm of female breast	10 374	4.1	25.4
8	Diseases of the urinary system	6987	2.8	10.4
9	Heart failure and complications and ill-defined heart disease	6536	2.6	9.3
10	Malignant neoplasm of colon, sigmoid, rectum and anus	6375	2.5	13.1
	All female deaths	253 286		

It is also possible to examine standardised mortality rates by social class and causes of death. For example, in the period 2001–2003, for men aged 25–64 in England and Wales, an almost clear gradient of increasing mortality is seen from moving down the social scale for five major causes of death shown in Table 1.5 for comparison. It can be seen that NS-SEC 1A and 1B have the lowest mortality. By contrast, those in routine occupations have death rates from these five causes that are between two and five times higher than those in managerial and professional jobs. A particular contrast is seen in deaths from suicide.

Leaving aside accidents and suicides for the next analysis, mortality rates for all cancers and all circulatory diseases for women show a similar trend. It is also possible to examine this trend across a north–south divide in England (Table 1.6). For example, age-standardised mortality rates for women aged 25–59 in the 2001–2003 period again show a gradient of increasing mortality in moving down the social scale (note the rates are expressed using a different denominator from the data in Table 1.5). There is also a clear difference according to geographical region, with higher rates reported consistently for northwest England compared with southwest England. Of course, many reasons have been suggested to explain the inequalities between region, including differences in unemployment risk, selective migration, concentrations of deprived areas and material disadvantage.

Table 1.5 Standard mortality rates per million according to National Statistics Socio-economic Classification and causes of death for men (25–64 years) in England and Wales between 2001 and 2003. (Data from White *et al.* 2008.)

NS-SEC analytical class	Ischaemic heart disease	Stroke	Cancer	Accidents	Suicide
1A Employers and managers in large organisations	410	76	806	79	47
1B Higher professionals	417	84	838	91	94
2. Lower managerial and professional occupations	563	118	990	103	111
3. Intermediate occupations	597	117	911	153	175
4. Small employers and own-account workers	663	147	1090	164	154
5. Lower supervisory and technical occupations	859	172	1402	148	136
6. Semi-routine occupations	1066	225	1469	251	243
7. Routine occupations	1193	230	1584	285	268

Table 1.6 Age-standardised mortality rates for selected causes and regions by National Statistics Socio-economic Classification for women (25–59) in 2001–2003. (Data from Langford *et al.* 2009.)

NS-SEC analytical class	All cancers (rates per 100 000)		All circulatory diseases (rates per 100 000)	
	Northwest	Southwest	Northwest	Southwest
1. Higher managerial and professional	69	76	18	11
2. Lower managerial and professional occupations	86	74	25	18
3. Intermediate occupations	76	65	29	22
4. Small employers and own-account workers	97	83	35	23
5. Lower supervisory and technical occupations	107	98	51	38
6. Semi-routine occupations	104	78	51	38
7. Routine occupations	125	112	78	49

Self-reported health

Patterns of life expectancy and mortality rates were referred to above, to demonstrate differences in health outcomes in the context of inequalities. This section examines self-reported health as a further indication of health inequalities, specifically in relation to ethnicity. In 2004 the Health Survey for England (Sproston and Mindell 2006) was rolled out specifically to update the government on knowledge about the health of ethnic minority groups; it focused on 'the seven largest minority ethnic groups in England', namely black Caribbean, black African, Indian, Pakistani, Bangladeshi, Chinese and Irish ethnic groups.

In summary, the survey found the highest prevalence of limiting long-standing illness (that affects their activities in any way) in Indian, Pakistani, Bangladeshi and Irish men and in black Caribbean and Pakistani and Bangladeshi women compared with the general population (Table 1.7). Conversely, Chinese and black African men and women were less likely than the general population, and all other groups, to report longstanding and limiting longstanding illness. In addition, Chinese, black African, Indian and Irish men and women were far less likely to report acute sickness than men and women in the general population and other ethnic minority groups.

As explained in the section above though, health inequalities are a result of a number of compounding factors and limiting longstanding illness is closely associated with both social class and household income. In the ethnic minority groups, in the main, people in the lowest income tertile had higher

Table 1.7 Standardised prevalence of self-reported limiting, longstanding illness in ethnic minority groups presented as standardised risk ratios. (Data from Sproston and Mindell 2006.)

Gender	Black Caribbean	Black African	Indian	Pakistani	Bangladeshi	Chinese	Irish	General population
Men	1.00	0.63	1.12	1.17	1.52	0.57	1.11	1
Women	1.20	0.83	0.86	1.60	1.22	0.46	0.80	1

Table 1.8 Standardised prevalence of self-reported limiting, longstanding illness in ethnic minority groups according to household income and gender. (Data from Sproston and Mindell 2006.)

Ethnicity	Equivalised household income tertile					
	Men			Women		
	Lowest	Middle	Highest	Lowest	Middle	Highest
Black Caribbean	1.109	0.849	0.667	1.173	1.013	0.812
Black African	0.651	0.751	0.489	0.72	0.559	0.673
Indian	1.223	0.958	0.604	0.805	0.717	0.69
Pakistani	1.133	0.8	0.379	1.19	1.241	0.939
Bangladeshi	1.037	0.813	0.353	0.978	0.917	1.410
Chinese	1.014	0.678	0.565	0.645	0.488	0.637
Irish	1.341	1.069	0.892	1.040	1.088	0.800
General population	1.13	1.062	0.934	1.097	1.109	0.888

age-adjusted risk ratios for limiting longstanding illness than those in the general population and those in the highest income tertile (Table 1.8).

The survey also enquired about the nature of people's illnesses. In the main, musculoskeletal conditions, followed by heart and circulatory problems, endocrine and metabolic disorders and diseases of the respiratory system were the most commonly reported longstanding illnesses. For conditions relating to the heart and circulatory system, risk ratios were generally above one among black Caribbean and South Asian (Indian, Pakistani, Bangladeshi) men and women and black African women. The risk ratio for musculoskeletal problems appeared to be high for Pakistani women and Irish men. For South Asian men and black Caribbean, Pakistani and Bangladeshi women, problems with the endocrine and the metabolic system are a common longstanding illness. Chinese men and women and black African men were less likely to report disorders of the musculoskeletal system than the general

Table 1.9 Standardised prevalence of bad or very bad self-assessed general health in ethnic minority groups expressed as standardised risk ratios. (Data from Sproston and Mindell 2006.)

Gender	Black Caribbean	Black African	Indian	Pakistani	Bangladeshi	Chinese	Irish	General population
Men	1.37	0.81	1.45	2.33	3.77	0.75	1.41	1
Women	1.90	1.68	1.39	3.54	4.02	0.55	0.74	1

population. In addition, black African men and women, and Indian and Chinese women were less likely to report disorders of the respiratory system than the general population.

In relation to self-assessed general health, Bangladeshi and Pakistani men and women, and black Caribbean women, reported substantially worse general health compared with the general population (Table 1.9). Chinese women were the only group much less likely to report bad or very bad health compared with the general population. Of course, similar to the general population, the majority of people reported good or very good health, so the figures do have to be taken in the context that a much lower proportion of people, including ethnic minorities, reported bad or very bad health overall. While the prevalence of bad or very bad self-reported health increased with age for the general population and all ethnic minority groups, this was particularly so with the Bangaldeshi and Pakistani groups. In terms of mental health and possible psychiatric morbidity, Bangladeshi men and Pakistani men and women were more likely than the general population to have a score indicative of possible psychiatric disorder.

The 2004 Health Survey for England (Sproston and Mindell 2006) also examined social support and found that prevalence of severe lack of social support was much higher among men and women in all minority ethnic groups, except Irish men and women. This was particularly marked among the Pakistani and Bangladeshi men and women. Reporting poor health can be strongly associated with use of health services and mortality. In the 1999 Health Survey for England (Erens *et al.* 2001) people were also asked about the use of health services. That survey found South Asian and black Caribbean men were more likely than the general population to have consulted their general practitioner in the previous two weeks and to have had more than one consultation over this period. Among women, contact rates were significantly higher for South Asian and Irish women. In terms of prescribed medication, the 2004 Health Survey for England found that, when comparing the risk ratios of taking four or more prescribed medicines across minority ethnic groups, most were around the same level as men and women in the general population. However, the exceptions were Pakistani and Bangladeshi women and, to a lesser extent, Indian men; these groups were more likely to be taking four or more prescribed medications than the general population.

The 1999 Health Survey for England (Erens *et al.* 2001) looked in detail at the types of medicines prescribed. In the general population, medication for cardiovascular diseases and diseases relating to the central nervous system (CNS), made up the most frequently-consumed types of medicines in both men and women. There was some variation in the ethnic minority groups. For example, Bangladeshi men and women were more likely to take medicines relating to the gastrointestinal system (GI), and South Asian women were two to three times more likely to take medication relating to nutrition and blood (e.g., because of higher rates of anaemia in South Asian women). Perhaps also of specific interest to pharmacists is that black Caribbean and South Asian men were two to three times more likely to be taking medication in relation to the endocrine system, with a third of medicines dispensed in this group being for diabetic control. Again, this is consistent with the higher prevalence of diabetes in this section of the population. Indian men and black Caribbean women had significantly higher cardiovascular-related prescribed medication than the general population, while Bangladeshi men had more CNS and musculoskeletal-related prescribed medication than the general population. Chinese men had significantly lower usage of CNS and musculoskeletal medication and Chinese women of CNS medication.

Health behaviours

Having examined life expectancy and mortality rates across a number of factors including gender, socioeconomic classification and geographical region and self-reported health (mainly in relation to ethnicity), this section examines patterns of health behaviours linked to morbidity and mortality. The pattern of behaviours examined here will include smoking, alcohol consumption, obesity and sexual health. This is because health behaviours are thought strongly to influence health outcomes, and behaviours can be associated with inequalities in society. But it is important to note that behaviours are not just driven by health inequalities – that would be too simplistic a view. Healthy or risky behaviour and therefore health outcomes are a result of the interaction between cultural, community and personal values and beliefs. Another note of caution relates to the fact that it is not only vulnerability to disease that is related to health behaviours. As discussed in Chapter 5, what people do when they experience ill health is also an important determinant of health outcomes.

Smoking is related to a number of respiratory cancers, and other respiratory diseases. The proportion of adult regular smokers in Great Britain fell in the decade to 2008 (Hughes 2010). Although in 1998 almost 30% of men

Table 1.10 Adult (more than 16 years) cigarette smoking habits by gender (%). (Data from Hughes 2010.)

	1998	2000	2001	2002	2003	2004	2005	2006	2007	2008
Men										
Current cigarette smoker	30	29	28	27	28	26	25	23	22	22
Ex-regular cigarette smoker	29	27	27	28	27	28	27	27	28	30
Never or only occasionally smoked	42	44	45	46	45	46	47	50	50	49
Women										
Current cigarette smoker	26	25	26	25	24	23	23	21	20	21
Ex-regular cigarette smoker	20	20	21	21	21	20	21	21	21	22
Never or only occasionally smoked	53	54	53	54	55	57	57	58	59	58

and 26% of women smoked on a regular basis, these proportions had fallen to 22% and 21%, respectively by 2008 (Table 1.10). This was matched with an increase in the proportion of people who had never or only occasionally smoked and the proportion of ex-smokers. In addition, in Great Britain in 2008 the highest proportion of smokers was in Scotland (23% of men and 24% of women), the lowest proportion of men smoking was in Wales (20%) and England had the lowest proportion of women smokers at 20%.

The 2004 Health Survey for England (Sproston and Mindell 2006) highlighted differences in the self-reported prevalence of cigarette smoking among men in ethnic minority groups compared with the general population; both Bangladeshi and Irish men were more likely to report currently smoking than the general population. Indian men were less likely to report currently smoking compared with the general population. Women from South Asian, Chinese and black African groups were significantly more likely than those in the general population to report never regularly smoking cigarettes.

Drinking alcohol is linked to a range of diseases such as cancer of the liver and cirrhosis of the liver. In spring 2011, the guidelines from the Chief Medical Officer for England suggested that consuming three to four units of alcohol per day for men and two to three units for women would not be expected to lead to significant health risks. The amounts are different because men's bodies can process alcohol more quickly than women's. Children of course are advised to steer clear of alcohol, certainly until they are 15 years of age. If young people between 15 and 17 years of age do drink alcohol, the

CMO's advice is that it should always be under the supervision of the parent or carer, should take place no more than once a week and for consumption to never exceed the recommended daily limits for adults.

However, in Great Britain in 2008 according to the General Lifestyle Survey conducted for the ONS (Robinson and Bugler 2010), 16% of men aged over 16 years drank double the recommended daily alcohol guideline at least once in the week prior to the interview, as did 15% of women (Table 1.11). A much higher proportion of men (21%) drank more than double the recommended units at least once in the previous week compared with women (14%). Only 63% of men and 71% of women drank within the recommended guidelines. Consuming more than double the recommended daily limit is defined as binge-drinking; the younger adult population were more likely to binge-drink. For example, 30% of 16–24 year old men and 24% of women in the same age group drank more than double the recommended daily allowance at least once in the previous week. In 2008, alcohol-related deaths had more than doubled compared with 1991 (9031 deaths vs 4144 deaths, respectively) with more alcohol-related deaths occurring in men (2532 in 1991 vs 5999 in 2008) compared with women (1612 in 1991 vs 3032 in 2008).

The 2004 Health Survey for England (Sproston and Mindell 2006) also highlighted differences in the self-reported consumption of alcohol among

Table 1.11 Consumption of alcohol by gender and age, according to the General Lifestyle Survey conducted in 2008 for the Office for National Statistics. (Data from Robinson and Bugler 2010.)

	Percentage of alcohol consumption in week before survey				
	16–24 years	25–44 years	45–65 years	65 years and over	All aged 16 years and over
Men					
Drank nothing in the previous week	37	28	26	34	30
Drank up to 4 units	21	30	33	44	33
Drank more than 4 units and up to 8 units	12	15	20	14	16
Drank more than 8 units	30	27	21	7	21
Women					
Drank nothing in the previous week	48	41	40	57	45
Drank up to 4 units	16	22	28	33	26
Drank more than 4 units and up to 8 units	12	16	19	8	15
Drank more than 8 units	24	20	13	2	14

men and women in ethnic minority groups compared with the general population. Men and women from all ethnic minority groups were less likely to drink alcohol and drank smaller amounts compared with the general population but this was not the case for the Irish who drank as frequently as the general population. In addition, ethnic groups were more likely than the general population to be non-drinkers, apart from the Irish who were as likely, with the highest percentage of non-drinkers found among Pakistani adults and Bangladeshi men and women.

Being obese is associated with a number of serious chronic diseases such as type 2 diabetes, hypertension and hyperlipidaemia, all of which are risk factors for cardiovascular diseases. In England in 2008, 36.9% of adults aged over 16 had a body mass index (BMI) that was considered overweight (Table 1.12). While this was a slight decrease compared with the proportion in 1994 (37.4%), sadly the proportion of adults classified as obese rose by 10 percentage points from 15.7% in 1994 to 24.5% in 2008 (Hughes 2010). A slightly higher proportion were classified as obese in Scotland in 2008 (26.8%) compared with a lower proportion of adults in Wales (21.0%). In addition, the proportion of morbidly obese adults doubled from 1% of the adult population in England in 1994 to 2% in 2008. The highest proportion of obese or overweight adults in England was in the 65–74 age range (77.1%) compared with 33.5% in the 16–24 age range. In Wales and Scotland, being overweight or obese was most prevalent in the 55–64 year olds (68.0% and 78.9%, respectively) and again least prevalent in the 16–24 age range (30.0% and 38.0%, respectively). Sadly the proportion of children under 16 classified as obese or overweight rose from 25% in 1995 to 30% in 2008 in England, with similar proportions in Wales (33%) and Scotland (32%).

The 2004 Health Survey for England (Sproston and Mindell 2006) had also highlighted differences in the weight of men and women in ethnic minority groups compared with the general population. Chinese and South Asian men were less likely to be overweight or obese than the general population

Table 1.12 Adult body mass index (%) according to the Health Survey for England. (Data from Hughes 2010.)

BMI	1994	1996	1998	2000	2002	2004	2006	2007	2008
Underweight (<18.5)	1.7	1.7	1.7	1.5	1.7	1.6	1.6	1.6	1.8
Normal (18.5 to <25)	45.2	42.2	40.6	38.6	37.7	36.7	36.8	37.7	36.8
Overweight (25 to <30)	37.4	38.7	38.3	38.8	38.1	38.8	37.6	36.7	36.9
Obese (30 and over) (i.e. includes morbidly obese)	15.7	17.5	19.4	21.2	22.5	22.9	23.9	24.0	24.5
Morbidly obese (40 and over)	1.0	0.9	1.3	1.5	1.8	1.7	2.1	1.8	2.0

whereas the likelihood of black African or Caribbean and Irish men being overweight or obese was the same as for men in the general population. For women, the likelihood of being overweight or obese was higher in black African, Caribbean and Pakistani women. Chinese women were half as likely to be overweight or obese as women in the general population.

Having unprotected sexual intercourse raises the risk of contracting sexually transmitted infections (STIs) such as human immunodeficiency virus (HIV), chlamydia and gonorrhoea. Injecting drug-users also run the risk of contracting HIV through sharing of injecting equipment. Substantial morbidity and mortality (HIV can lead to acquired immunodeficiency syndrome, AIDS) are associated with HIV and other STIs and the impact of disease falls disproportionately on marginalised populations, including men who have sexual intercourse with other men and some black and minority ethnic groups. The incidence of STIs can be tracked by examining consultations at genitourinary medicine clinics. The number of new STI episodes rose between 2001 and 2008, with chlamydia presenting as the most prevalent STI in 2008 (over 123 000 new cases) (Hughes 2010). Syphilis has the lowest prevalence among the STIs yet cases rose by more than 18 times from 1998 to 2008 (from 139 to 2524 cases). Men accounted for 67% of new episodes of gonorrhoea, 89% of syphilis and 53% of genital warts, whereas new episodes of genital herpes were more common among women, accounting for 61% of new cases. In terms of HIV, the rate of new HIV diagnoses was 109.2 per million population in the UK in 2008, nearly double that in 1985 (66.5 per million), although this rate is still lower than a peak in 2004 (148 per million). The diagnoses of HIV is highest in England (120.1 per million population) compared with Wales (44.4 per million), Scotland (58.0 per million) and Northern Ireland (51.8 per million).

Men who have sexual intercourse with other men are the behavioural group at the highest risk of acquiring HIV. In 2005, the Health Protection Agency reported this group accounting for one third (2356/7450) of new HIV diagnoses in the UK, while making up nearly half of all diagnoses since 1981 (36 531/78 938) (UK Collaborative Group for HIV and STI Surveillance 2006). It also estimated the percentage of populations living with diagnosed HIV by ethnic group to be as follows. In those aged 15–59 of Indian, Pakistani or Bangladeshi origin, 0.03% were estimated to be living with HIV, while the figures were 0.08% for those considered 'white', 0.3% for black Caribbean people and 3.6% for black Africans. The figures reflected the new diagnoses of HIV that year, when nearly two thirds (3691/5902) of all new diagnoses of HIV in England, Wales and Northern Ireland were among the black and minority ethnic individuals. In this subgroup, 83% of new diagnoses (3064) were among black Africans, 6.0% were among black Caribbeans (206), 2.1% among those of Indian, Pakistani or Bangladeshi origin (77) and the remainder (344) among other or mixed ethnicities.

Policy recommendations and pharmacy

The conditions most strongly associated with health inequalities are cancer and cardiovascular diseases. These in turn are associated with smoking, alcohol and drug use and obesity. Thus one of the key recommendations arising from the Marmot Review examining health inequalities in England relates to changing health behaviours. Changing health behaviours are of course normally associated with the concepts of ill-health prevention and health promotion. The WHO Ottawa Charter for Health Promotion (1986) defined health promotion as 'the process of enabling people to increase control over, and to improve their health'. Other wide-ranging definitions of these concepts also exist. In England a broader definition of ill-health prevention sees this as 'a clinical, social, behavioural, educational, environmental, fiscal or legislative intervention or broad partnership programme designed to reduce the risk of mental and physical illness, disability or premature death and/or to promote long-term physical, social, emotional and psychological wellbeing'. The Marmot Review uses this definition to highlight the importance of viewing ill-health prevention and health promotion as a shared responsibility across a range of sectors and services and not just a domain of the National Health Service.

Nonetheless, in terms of the NHS, the Marmot Review recommends the implementation of evidence-based programmes of ill-health prevention such as those focused on smoking cessation, alcohol reduction and weight loss (Marmot et al. 2010). Interestingly, the Marmot Review also notes that pharmacists are among a range of primary care health professionals who do not see tackling social determinants of health inequalities as core business (Marmot et al. 2010). It recommends prioritisation of health inequalities as a routine part of primary care so that this can be reflected in contracts with independent contractors such as pharmacists. Indeed, in spring 2011, the community pharmacy contract in England included a number of services related directly to public health activities (PSNC 2011). 'Essential Services' included an obligatory role in the 'Promotion of Healthy Lifestyles', while 'Enhanced and Local Services' (which are determined and negotiated locally) included 'Needle and Syringe Exchange', 'Stop Smoking', 'Chlamydia Screening and Treatment', 'Emergency Hormonal Contraception', as well as medicine-related services such as minor ailments, medication reviews, supplementary prescribing and services for care homes. In addition, the pharmacy contract includes 'Advanced Services', which include the 'Medicines Use Review and Prescription Intervention Service' as well as a (new for 2011) 'New Medicines Service'. It could be argued that quite a number of the services outlined in the pharmacy contract in England attempt to address health behaviours via the pharmacy at a one-to-one level of interaction, be it in relation to ill-health prevention or (as yet to be elaborated on in this book) improving medication-related health behaviours.

Conclusion

A rationale for studying social and cognitive pharmacy has been provided; social and psychosocial factors impact on behaviour to a great extent, strongly influencing people's health and illness-related outcomes. To provide evidence, health inequalities and people's experiences of health according to various social determinants have been examined, rather comprehensively. In the process, the types of health outcomes data that demonstrate these health inequalities have been considered. The health conditions most strongly associated with health inequalities are cancer and cardiovascular diseases, which in turn are associated with smoking, alcohol and drug use and obesity. Thus one of the key recommendations for addressing health inequalities relates to changing health behaviours, which can be tackled through knowledge of psychology. The main aim of the remainder of the theory chapters is therefore to provide relevant psychological know-how to equip pharmacists with the tools required to influence their patients' health and illness-related behaviour at the individual level. Most of this psychological knowledge arises from research. Thus to empower readers with an ability to critically examine the theory later presented, Chapter 2 begins with a detailed examination of the methods that lead to the generation of pharmacy-related social and psychological knowledge, before moving on to consider theories and methods related to behaviour change in more detail from Chapter 3 onwards.

Sample examination questions

Students may wish to use the following sample questions to aid their learning and revision before examinations:

1   Describe the social determinants of health.

2   Define risky health behaviours using examples to illustrate your answer.

3   Indicate the importance of the bio-psychosocial approach to health.

4   Demonstrate the importance of one social determinant of health to pharmacy.

5   Justify the learning and teaching of social and cognitive pharmacy at degree level.

6 To what extent are social factors such as class and ethnicity of relevance to pharmacy?

7 Defend the position that pharmacists should be taught only biomedical knowledge rather than social or cognitive pharmacy.

References and further reading

Acheson D (1998). *Independent Inquiry into Inequalities in Health* (The Acheson Report). London: The Stationery Office.

Ashton K, Kent K (2008). Annual population survey household data sets. *Economic & Labour Market Review (ONS publication)*, 2(10): 44–51.

Braveman P *et al.* (2011). The social determinants of health: Coming of age. *Annual Review of Public Health*, **32**: 381–398. doi: 10.1146/annurev-publhealth-031210-101218.

Commission on Social Determinants of Health (2008). *Closing the Gap in a Generation: Health Equity through Action on the Social Determinants of Health* (Final report of the Commission on Social Determinants of Health). Geneva: World Health Organization.

Department of Health and Social Security (1980). *Inequalities in Health: Report of a Research Working Group* (The Black Report). London: DHSS.

Dobbs J *et al.* eds. (2006). *Focus on Ethnicity and Religion* (ONS publication). Basingstoke, Hants: Palgrave Macmillan.

Erens B *et al.* eds. (2001). *Health Survey for England: The Health of Minority Ethnic Groups 1999*. London: Joint Health Surveys Unit.

Hall C (2006). *A Picture of the United Kingdom using the National Statistics Socioeconomic Classification*. London: Office for National Statistics.

Horne R *et al.* (1999). The beliefs about medicines questionnaire: The development and evaluation of a new method for assessing the cognitive representation of medication. *Psychology and Health*, **14**: 1–24.

Hughes M ed. (2010). *Social Trends 40*. London: Office for National Statistics.

Langford A *et al.* (2009). Social inequalities in female mortality by region and by selected causes of death, England and Wales, 2001–03. *Health Statistics Quarterly (ONS publication)*, **44**: 7–26.

Marmot MG *et al.* on behalf of the Marmot Review (2010). *Fair Society, Healthy Lives: Strategic Review of Health Inequalities in England post-2010*. London: Department of Health.

Matthews KA, Gallo LC (2011). Psychological perspectives on pathways linking socioeconomic status and physical health. *Annual Review of Psychology*, **62**: 501–530.

Miller G *et al.* (2009). Health psychology: Developing biologically plausible models linking the social world and physical health. *Annual Review of Psychology*, **60**: 501–524.

Office for National Statistics (2005). *The National Statistics Socioeconomic Classification (NS-SEC): User Manual*. Basingstoke, Hants: Palgrave Macmillan.

Office for National Statistics (2010a). Life expectancy at birth and at age 65 by local areas in the United Kingdom, 2007–09. *Statistical Bulletin*. London: ONS.

Office for National Statistics (2010b). Death registrations by cause in England and Wales, 2009. *Statistical Bulletin*. London: ONS.

Ottawa Charter for Health Promotion (1986). WHO/HPR/HEP/95.1. World Health Organization: Geneva.

Pharmaceutical Services Negotiating Committee (PSNC) (2011). *The Pharmacy Contract*. URL: http://www.psnc.org.uk/pages/introduction.html (accessed 4 August 2011).

Robinson S, Bugler C (2010). *Smoking and Drinking Among Adults: General Lifestyle Survey 2008*. London: Office for National Statistics.

Sproston K, Mindell J eds. (2006). *Health Survey for England 2004: The health of minority ethnic groups*. Leeds: The Information Centre.

UK Collaborative Group for HIV and STI Surveillance (2006). *A Complex Picture. HIV and other sexually transmitted infections in the United Kingdom: 2006.* London: Health Protection Agency, Centre for Infections.

Umberson D *et al.* (2010). Social relationships and health behavior across the life course. *Annual Review of Sociology,* **36:** 139–157.

White C *et al.* (2008). Social inequalities in male mortality for selected causes of death by the National Statistics Socioeconomic Classification, England and Wales, 2001–2003. *Health Statistics Quarterly* (ONS publication), **38:** 19–32.

Wilkinson R, Pickett K (2010). *The Spirit Level: Why Equality is Better for Everyone.* London: Penguin.

World Health Organization (1948). *WHO Constitution.* Geneva: WHO.

2

Generation of pharmacy-related sociological and psychological knowledge

Synopsis

This chapter gives an overview of the key points relating to the methods that inform sociology and psychology research in relation to pharmacy practice. The chapter explains the manner in which sociological and psychological knowledge is generated through theorising and research. It explains differences between the philosophical standpoints of empiricism and interpretation, relating these to quantitative and qualitative methodology, respectively. The aim is to introduce the rationale for conducting different types of research. The chapter also describes features of quantitative and qualitative data analysis. A key feature of this chapter is the practical use of examples to explain the role of research in generating knowledge in pharmacy. Gaining an understanding of the basis of different research methodology should later facilitate independent scrutiny of the worth and value of pharmacy-related social and psychological theory and knowledge generated through research.

Learning outcomes

You should be able to demonstrate knowledge and understanding of the following after working through this chapter:

- the relationship between sociology, psychology and pharmacy research
- opposing philosophical positions taken within these fields
- key research approaches used within the disciplines of pharmaceutical sociology and psychology

- types of pharmaceutical sociology and psychology data generated through research and how they are generally analysed.

Introduction

Whether relating sociology or psychology (or both) to pharmacy, to be effective and credible, pharmaceutical sociologists and psychologists must keep up with and reflect evolving societies and human behaviour, and this is normally carried out through research. Research generates new information, which not only enriches existing knowledge but leads to further research in an iterative process. According to the *Oxford English Dictionary*, research is the systematic investigation into and study of materials and sources to establish facts and reach new conclusions. In broad terms, sociological and psychological research starts with a question or problem that needs to be investigated. The question or problem, preferably framed with reference to existing theories, is then narrowed to enable effective examination of it in a methodical manner. Once formulated in this way, the researcher can consider the types of data that would yield suitable information and the methods that would be appropriate to use in an attempt to answer the research question. After the data have been collected, and for some types of research in the course of data collection, the researcher can start analysing the information gathered for patterns that can be turned into evidence in the form of study results. Effective researchers then evaluate this evidence, where possible developing a theory or formulating other research questions to instigate the cycle of enquiry all over again.

Research is also a social institution in its own right, with a fixed set of norms and expectations attached to it (Abercrombi *et al.* 2000). Ultimately sociological and psychological research involves the collection, exploration and reporting of information about people and societies. However, what is considered acceptable research within these fields is often influenced by philosophical standpoints of the prevailing research communities. All knowledge is situated in a specific historical and social location and approaches to the construction of sociological and psychological knowledge are not exempt from this. In fact, establishing the location of psychosocial knowledge helps researchers make informed judgements about which methods and assumptions are most appropriate for their own research.

Exploring the concept: research methods

Let us return to a previous example and imagine wanting to find out more about independent prescribing. The first step would be to define the research question or describe the problem in a way that lends itself to investigation. What is it about independent prescribing that needs to be investigated? Based on preliminary evidence, the researcher may want to test the premise that independent prescribing status has not been taken up by pharmacists to the same degree across Strategic Health Authorities (SHAs). Alternatively, the researcher may want to investigate doctors' understanding of non-medical prescribing and the meaning they attach to pharmacists taking up this new role. These research questions would lend themselves to different styles of research. To answer the first question, the researcher would be likely to collect quantitative data relating to numbers of independent pharmacist prescribers, numbers of registered pharmacists and so on in different SHAs. To answer the second question, the researcher is more likely to collect qualitative data relating to doctors' opinions and experiences of pharmacist prescribing. Whatever type of data is collected, the researcher would use the conventional methods of analysis for that data type to yield study results, which they would then put into perspective in relation to existing theories and research. For example, a finding that indeed the uptake of independent prescribing by pharmacists varies across SHAs would be related to previous findings, say by other researchers or in relation to the uptake of the related activity of supplementary prescribing by pharmacists. The two approaches to data collection, namely quantitative and qualitative research, are the topic of the section on page 43, which considers each approach in detail.

Two important philosophical standpoints within pharmaceutically relevant sociology and psychology research

As mentioned above, the process of creating sociological and psychological knowledge relates to ideas about what constitutes appropriate research within a particular philosophical perspective. This section will focus on explaining the basic assumptions of empiricism versus interpretation as two philosophical approaches to research because both offer good justification for the way in which most pharmacy-related psychosocial research is conducted. In brief, while the tradition of empiricism is concerned with the creation of objective data, interpretation relates to the analysis of meaning in subjective accounts. These concepts lead to methodological differences in the conduct of research (Yates 2004). With empiricism, but not exclusively, nomothetic approaches use quantitative methodology to study and create generally applicable models and scientific laws. With interpretation, again not necessarily exclusively, idiographic approaches use qualitative methodology to study and depict individual or specific circumstances without the need for generalisation. Debates about different ways in which data are gathered and used in research relate to epistemology. Epistemology is the theory of knowledge, of how we know what we know, especially the analysis of what should count as knowledge, the validity of knowledge, what distinguishes belief from knowledge, the kinds of things that are to be known, and indeed whether anything can be known for certain. Epistemology, which is linked to ontology (see below), drives the research methodology, and ultimately the data generated (Fig. 2.1).

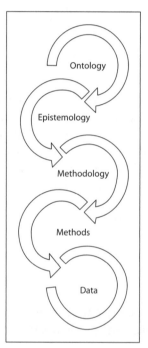

Figure 2.1 Ideas about what it means to be human (ontology), how we know what we know (epistemology), drives the rationale for the research (methodology) and ultimately the research methods and type of data generated.

Exploring the concept: epistemology

Let's use an example from everyday life, something that appears relatively straightforward, such as the driving test. In the UK, aspiring car drivers must pass a driving test before being allowed to take sole charge of a vehicle on public roads. This driving test involves both a practical component and a theoretical test, which nowadays includes an interactive hazard perception test. But up until 1996, the driving test was a practical assessment only. So why was the theoretical test introduced? And what does the hazard perception test (introduced in 2002) add to the arrangement? These questions are about the basis of what should count as a valid test of fitness-to-drive, in the vein of epistemological concerns. The other noteworthy point is about the nature of the data generated by the current driving test, which is designed to produce objective information within generally applicable models not dissimilar to the nomothetic approach to research. But what if the examiner was interested instead in studying and depicting the driver's understanding of driving and the meanings he or she attaches to the process? What if the examiner was not interested in using the data to score against acceptable performance criteria but wanted to find out more about the in-depth experiences of the driver? This approach would not be too dissimilar to the idiographic approach to research. Although an unlikely option for a driving test, with advancements in vehicle design, changing attitudes to road safety and countless other cultural developments, this second approach could provide some very useful information to keep the driving test valid and in itself fit-for-purpose. The introduction of the theory test and the hazard perception test would have come about for exactly these reasons.

The empiricist tradition

The ideas of those who follow the empiricist tradition are related to positivism, which asserts that science can provide an objective, value-free picture of the world. In this way it is helpful to understand the six interrelated assumptions that underline the positivist approach to the creation of knowledge (Yates 2004) (Fig. 2.2).

The first of these assumptions is that of naturalism that asserts it is possible to transfer the methods of the natural sciences (e.g., chemistry, physics) to the study of people and social structures within closed systems.

The second assumption is that of phenomenalism that asserts only knowledge gained through the physical senses exists, so that other concepts (e.g., 'compassion') become merely ideas that exist in people's minds.

The third is that of nominalism that asserts concepts not directly experienced through the senses are meaningless, so that abstract concepts (e.g., 'fairness') become merely names without corresponding reality.

Fourth is that of atomism, which asserts that objects of scientific study are interpretable through analysis into distinct and discrete elementary com-

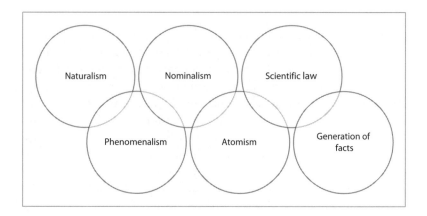

Figure 2.2 The six interrelated assumptions that underline the positivist approach to the creation of knowledge. (Data from Yates 2004.)

ponents. A simple pharmacy example is to think of the most discrete unit as an individual involved in an interaction in a dispensary and think of the situation as no more than a collection of individuals.

Fifth is that of the scientific law that asserts the purpose of research is to develop laws that explain empirical regularities occurring in different places and at different times (i.e., are generalisable). One may look for empirical regularities, for example, between numbers of dispensed items, numbers of support staff, hours worked and dispensing errors.

The sixth assumption is that relating to facts (rather than values), which asserts that only facts that can be verified through observational reference can be regarded as scientific, and that values cannot be because their verification will involve subjective assessment rather than observation and measurement. For example, a measure of the number of compounding errors in a pharmacy aseptic unit can be viewed as a fact, whereas the statement that aseptic units are soulless environments in which to work is a value statement.

Empiricism uses the notion that it is possible to study people and social structures 'scientifically' within closed systems. This idea can also be understood by reflecting on the experimental laboratory method, where a limited number of variables are identified, their behaviour and interrelationship observed while accounting for or avoiding interference from external (confounding) variables, to generate causal laws. The application of these assumptions to psychosocial research thus necessitates the identification of a limited number of measurable variables (whose properties are taken at face value), while excluding other possible influences, for the discovery and prediction of clear relationships to create generalisable laws. Data take a defined, quantifiable and objective form.

Exploring the concept: the empiricist tradition

Let's use an example to explore the application of these assumptions to pharmacy practice research. Imagine we are interested in studying the supply of weight-loss products in the pharmacy within the empiricist tradition. According to the above text, the first step would be to identify a limited number of variables to study. If we believe, for example, that there may be a relationship between the body mass index (BMI) and gender of people purchasing weight-loss products in pharmacies, we could set out to measure those two variables and their interrelationship in a carefully selected and representative sample of pharmacies. We would need to conduct the research in such a way that would enable generalisation of the findings to pharmacies per se in the future. We would also need to consider if the relationship between BMI and gender is influenced by other factors such as the geographical location of the pharmacy, the socioeconomic circumstances of the people purchasing the weight-loss products, or the type of pharmacy surveyed. Our research would need to account for or avoid interference from such external (confounding) variables. When we have conducted a sufficient number of measurements, we would explore the relationship between BMI and gender using statistical techniques that would account for the confounding variables. Let's imagine we find that overall there is a statistically significant difference in the mean BMI of male versus female clients with men who purchase weight-loss products in the pharmacy more likely to have a higher BMI compared with women. Within the empiricist tradition, we would use the study findings to produce statements of fact to relate the research more widely to pharmacies in general.

The interpretivist tradition

Those who follow interpretivist practices might argue that people and social life are too complex to be studied in simple closed systems as described above, at least in some instances. Far from being straightforward, social objects have intrinsic properties and a complexity that can interfere with the assumptions made by empiricist researchers (Yates 2004) (Fig. 2.3). The interpretative approach is based on the notion that people and social structures exist in open systems and should be studied instead to explore their interactions and subjectivity. Interpretivist researchers acknowledge the complexity of their objects of analysis and their interrelationship, assume no external boundary, and recognise that intrinsic properties and structures can interfere with results in countless ways so that future outcomes cannot

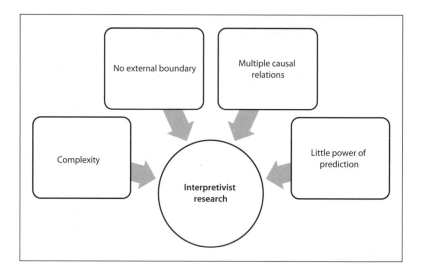

Figure 2.3   Some features that underline the interpretivist approach to the creation of knowledge. Data from Yates (2004).

be predicted with any degree of certainty. What is studied therefore is not standardised and measured but relates to people's experiences and thoughts, which are explored for their qualitative nature. Data take a descriptive and subjective form.

Exploring the concept: the interpretivist approach

Let's continue with the example involving the supply of weight-loss products purchased in the pharmacy. Those who follow interpretivist practices may argue that the relationship between BMI and gender of people purchasing weight-loss products in pharmacies is too complex to be studied in a quantitative and generalisable manner, even with the three confounding variables measured and considered. We imagined finding that men who purchase weight-loss products in the pharmacy were more likely to have a higher BMI compared with women in the example above. But is such an empirical regularity sufficient for establishing a causal law? What other explanations could there be for such an outcome? What were people's reasons for purchasing weight-loss products in the first place; what were their values and systems of belief? Following the interpretivist tradition, we may be more interested in studying individual circumstances to create an understanding of people's behaviour instead. We may be more interested to discover the meanings people attach to their purchase of the weight-loss products in the pharmacy. Imagine some people articulate that support from their regular partner contributed to their recent purchase of the product while others speak of longstanding attempts to tackle their weight through products available in the pharmacy, some talk about diet and exercise plans and others about recent health promotion campaigns, some people speak about referrals from their GP while others talk about positive experiences with pharmacy products in the past. If we acknowledge the importance of meaning in generating knowledge, the finding that men who purchase weight-loss products in the pharmacy were more likely to have a higher BMI compared with women as a principal finding seems no longer valid for our purpose.

Quantitative versus qualitative research methods

The empiricist versus interpretivist perspectives then lend themselves to different viewpoints in terms of the way in which knowledge can be created. While empiricism is concerned with studying or discovering general scientific laws, using the nomothetic approach to build testable theories that will yield universally relevant laws, interpretation is concerned with the detailed examination or discovery of particular situations and processes, using the idiographic approach to study individuals in depth and one at a time without the need for generalising. The overall idea though is that the set of methods used to answer a research question and the type of data generated should align with the theoretical perspective taken. Methodology is concerned with choosing the methods that are appropriate to the research question, to generate data that can be converted into the appropriate scientific evidence. In other words, it should be possible for a researcher to provide a rationale for the conduct of their enquiries based on their theoretical position. The nomothetic and idiographic approaches have also been understood in terms of quantitative versus qualitative research. Different methods will be used depending on whether the aim is to collect objective or subjective data, within the empiricist versus interpretivist traditions, respectively. A summary is provided here but those interested in learning more about research methods are directed towards an excellent book by Coolican (2009), which details a range of methods and analyses used in psychological research, applicable to a range of psychosocial pharmacy practice research. The *BMJ* also has a series of practice articles on research (2008), listed at the end of this chapter.

Quantitative methods, generally speaking, will yield objective data while qualitative methods will yield subjective data. Research that uses quantitative methods aims to establish general laws or statements that apply across different participants at different times. Therefore the entire mechanism of research including the study design, the nature of the data and the manner in which data are collected must all lend themselves to objectivity. What is more, the researchers must set out to collect the data in an impartial manner, to exclude their own personal values and biases. Specific techniques include establishing the research hypothesis at the outset of the study and consistency in data collection, for example, through the use of standardised instruments. As the aim is to produce generalisable data, quantitative research must also be replicable in that it should be possible for the study to be repeated with another sample at a different time and still produce similar results. Two specific methods used to create objective pharmacy-related psychosocial knowledge within the empiricist tradition are surveys and experiments.

Research that uses qualitative methods aims to capture the subjective nature of phenomena for assigned meanings and explanations, often through the analysis of language. Therefore the mechanism of qualitative research must enable the researcher to relate with the field of study to uncover how the people studied are creating, and being created by, their understandings of the world. An important element of qualitative research is that it need not follow distinct, predetermined stages, allowing researchers to move back and forth between research questions, collecting and analysing data in an iterative process. As well as creating an understanding of people's inner experiences, researchers who study subjectivities and meanings may wish to compare their results between different groups of people. To allow such comparisons, some form of simplification of data may be carried out, for example, by establishing common categories or themes in the data. Qualitative research can involve a range of data collection methods and approaches to data analysis. The creation of pharmacy-related data within the interpretative tradition can involve ethnographic methods (interviews, focus groups and observations) and discourse analysis of printed text.

Fundamentals of quantitative psychosocial research

Quantitative psychosocial research typically involves generating a theory and forming a research hypothesis, operationalising the concept, identifying target participants, setting up the study and collecting the data, analysing them and reporting on the findings. There should be a theoretical basis to all quantitative pharmacy-related sociology and psychology research. The theory utilised can relate to well-established knowledge (e.g., functionalism) or smaller, more specific ideas derived from previous research findings and models (e.g., adherence to medication). Say a researcher is interested in how patients' adherence to medicines can be improved; this will become their research question. However, clearly the question is too large to be tested in a single survey or experiment. Recall that research within the empiricist tradition necessitates the identification of a limited number of measurable variables for the discovery and prediction of clear relationships to create generalisable laws. So the quantitative researcher must identify a small measurable element of the theory for investigation. For example, the researcher may stipulate that receiving reminders via text messaging will improve adherence to medicines in young patients on short-term antibiotic treatment. This type of formal statement, predicting a relationship between the two entities (variables) of text message reminders and adherence to medication, is a research hypothesis. A detailed discussion of statistics is outside the scope of this book but for statistical reasons it is the null hypothesis that is tested in quantitative research. The null hypothesis would state there is no relationship between the two variables being studied, in this case between text message reminders and adherence to medication, and that any observed relationship is due to sampling error. But how can the variables text message reminders and adherence to medication be defined and measured in an objective way?

The concepts of text message reminders and adherence will need to be converted into more workable forms if they are to be measured objectively. The next step in quantitative research involves operationalising the research concepts to make them researchable. There needs to be a well-defined and simple way of administering and measuring the text message reminders and evaluating adherence to medication. For example, the researcher may devise standardised wording to send by phone to patients in the intervention group during a defined time period at predetermined intervals. By the same token, the researcher will need to devise a simple index to yield numerical data about adherence, starting with an exact definition of adherence in line with other acceptable descriptions. For example, adherence may be defined as the extent to which a patient acts in accordance with the dose and prescribed time points of a particular medication regimen. From there, the researcher may define the unit of measure for adherence as doses taken correctly per defined period of time, reported as proportion of prescribed doses taken at the prescribed time points. The researcher would of course also need to use a standardised tool for collecting this information to enable accurate, objective recording of the data, for example, through observation, patient self-reporting or more sophisticated means using electronic monitoring technology.

Measuring adherence is notoriously difficult and the researcher must consider at least the validity and reliability of the data collection instrument. Validity is the extent to which a measurement tool or questionnaire actually measures what it claims to be measuring. For example, where the researcher decides to use an electronic monitoring device that makes a recording every time the patient opens a tablet bottle, validity concerns such questions as whether the data generated actually relate to the patient's ingestion of the medicine (and therefore, adherence) or the mere opening of the bottle's lid. Reliability is the extent to which the tool gives reproducible results for an individual over time and comparable conditions. If the researcher decides to administer a questionnaire for self-reporting by patients, reliability concerns such questions as whether the instrument will return reproducible results time and again.

Another concern in quantitative psychosocial research is the selection of participants or respondents. Researchers working within the empiricist tradition must commit to finding a sufficient number of relevant participants to investigate in their studies. Quantitative researchers will normally use a sample of people drawn from the population under investigation, rather than researching the *entire* population; research with a large population is unlikely to be realistic, not least for reasons of practicability and cost. However, because research within the empiricist tradition aims to produce generalisable findings, the sample investigated should be representative of the population. After all, the analysis of information gained from the smaller sample will be used to make inferences about the larger population, the actual group of people to whom the findings will apply.

A number of sampling techniques exist. A detailed discussion of sampling methodology is outside of the scope of this book, nonetheless sampling methods can be classified as broadly fitting one of two categories of probability versus purposive sampling. Probability sampling methods concern the random selection of individuals from the target population where each individual has a known chance of being selected. Examples include simple random, systematic sample, stratified/structured random and cluster sample methods. Purposive sampling methods concern the selection of research participants based on their characteristics rather than at random. Examples include homogeneous sample, snowball and convenience sample methods. The decision about which sampling method to use is dependent on statistical as well as practical reasons but quantitative researchers should aim ultimately to minimise any bias that can lead to the selection of an unrepresentative sample.

Surveys and experiments are the two most common study designs used to create pharmacy-related psychosocial knowledge within the empiricist tradition. Although pharmacy practice researchers also make use of audits as investigative tools, audits are not *research* and fall outside of the scope of this section. This is because, although they serve a useful purpose in their own right, audits will aim to collect numerical data only to generate a snapshot view of actual practice against set standards without the need for creating causal explanations. Experiments and surveys, on the other hand, will involve the systematic collection of quantifiable data for the primary purpose of making inferences about the results. Both methods share the need to use statistical testing to address the research hypothesis, i.e., to analyse the relationship between two or more variables measured through the research.

Generally speaking, experiments, which normally involve the measurement of participants' behaviour, are more likely to be favoured by those working within the realm of psychology and surveys, which normally involve asking participants to answer a series of questions, by those working within sociology. Researchers use experiments to create situations in which a limited number of factors can be manipulated and their effects on the participants measured, against a 'control' group (where the factors are not manipulated). Recall the study described above, which aimed to measure the impact of text messaging on adherence. The researchers could choose to send text message reminders to the intervention group, with no reminders to the control group, and then measure adherence to medicines in order to make inferences about the effect of the reminders on adherence. Surveys do not involve manipulating any variables but instead involve collecting data from participants about all variables and then analysing any interrelationship between the variables. For example, researchers interested in examining people's attitudes towards non-prescription medicines may set out to measure sociodemographic characteristics of survey respondents as well as their tendency to seek information from the pharmacist, hypothesising a relationship between the two.

Inferential statistics can be used to measure the differences described above and the use of a number of such tests will be discussed. Before that, an important concept known as sampling error must be considered. Imagine a difference is found between groups of participants/respondents. For example, there may be a difference in adherence rates in the intervention versus control groups in the experiment or there may be a difference in the frequency with which men versus women seek pharmacists' advice, as revealed in the survey. There is a possibility that such findings may represent a real difference between the groups in the wider population or the findings may be a product of sampling error. Recall that in conducting quantitative psychosocial research investigators are impelled to use 'samples' of populations to make estimates about those populations, rather than using the entire population. Despite attempts at obtaining a representative sample, it is still possible for data relating to the sample to be different from that of the population. For example, women's tendency to seek information from the pharmacist may be different in the sample surveyed compared with the broader population of women. That is, the mean and the standard deviation of the results from the study may be different from the mean and standard deviation of results for the entire population (if this could be measured).

Increasing the sample size is likely to bring the mean and standard deviation of the results closer to that of the population. It is also possible to estimate the 'population mean' from mean and standard deviation values of a sample. Once this is calculated, using confidence intervals, it should be possible to compare the means obtained from two samples and work out if they are sufficiently different to be data from two different populations.

For example, it should be possible to compare the mean adherence score from the intervention group in the experiment described above with the mean adherence score from the control group to determine if the groups are sufficiently different because of an effect caused by the text message reminders, or whether the difference is simply due to sampling error. Similarly, it should be possible to compare the mean frequency with which women seek pharmacists' advice with the mean frequency with which men seek pharmacists' advice, and determine if the results for men versus women are sufficiently different because of a real relationship between gender and information-seeking behaviour, or whether the difference is simply due to sampling error. Confidence intervals can be calculated using standard statistical software packages such as SPSS. It is normal practice to calculate a 95% confidence interval. The 95% confidence interval for a sample mean is the range of values within which the population mean may fall (with 95% certainty) and is normally expressed as the lower bound and the upper bound representing the limits.

The analyses of data gathered via the experimental or survey methods are likely to involve the use of inferential statistical tests. Inferential statistics use laws of probability to make inferences about a population based on information from a sample. A number of inferential statistics exist for normally distributed data including t-tests, analysis of variance (ANOVA), chi-square, and regression analysis, which are all parametric tests. Although a detailed discussion of statistical tests falls outside of the scope of this book, it is important to emphasise that researchers follow a rationale when selecting which test to use. One of the factors that influences researchers in test selection is whether a *relationship* or a *difference* is being sought. Another is the nature of the data collected, for example, whether data are categorical or continuous. Yet another consideration is the nature of the study, for example, whether an experiment, or a correlation or association study, and indeed the number and type of variables involved. A simple rule-of-thumb is that experimental studies, looking for differences between two or more conditions but measuring parametric data on a continuous scale, will use either the t-test or ANOVA. By contrast, studies that involve two categorical variables will use the chi-square test and those that involve two continuous variables will use Pearson correlation.

Fundamentals of qualitative psychosocial research

Qualitative psychosocial research typically involves generating a research question instead of a research hypothesis. This is because the researchers are more likely to be interested in an exploration of the subjective and broader social meanings that people attach to their thoughts and actions. For example, a research question might relate to the experience of patients engaging in the Medicines Use Review (MUR) service. Researchers using qualitative methods might access a range of material that will give deeper and richer insights into people, the social contexts and social practices. For example, researchers might interview patients and pharmacists engaging in the MUR, they might examine the written records of completed MURs and they might also examine booking arrangements and patient literature relating to the MUR.

Another term to consider at this stage is *ontology*, the theory of the nature of existence or what it is to be human. Some researchers believe that humans are social beings who create themselves and are shaped by their understanding of the world around them via language and communication. This is important because belief about what it is to be a person will shape belief about what constitutes knowledge, so ontology is closely linked to epistemology and therefore methodology. Remembering that epistemology concerns 'how we know what we know' and methodology concerns the overall theoretical rationale that underpins a research question, all these positions then influence a set of methods and therefore the generation of specific types of data. Perspectives operating within the interpretivist tradition favour qualitative approaches, where human thought and action is interpreted by focusing on understandings held and articulated by the research participants, and to some extent the researchers themselves. Although data collection methods in themselves cannot be strictly 'qualitative', the following methods are normally associated with the generation of qualitative data: semi- or unstructured interviews, participant and non-participant observation, group discussions and interviews and the analysis of documentary materials.

Qualitative research methods are not described in detail here but it is important to emphasise that, whatever methods are adopted, they must relate to the theoretical framework, the topic area and the research question. Just as the research methods will vary according to the researchers' aims, so will methods of data interpretation. The focus of this section is to present a general overview of some qualitative methods of interpretation used in pharmacy practice research; namely, grounded theory, thematic analysis and discourse analysis.

Grounded theory

Grounded theory relies on the analysis of text (Glaser and Strauss 1967). In a pure form, this is an inductive process of analysis that derives theory from the data themselves so that theory is 'grounded' in the qualitative data from which it is developed. Using grounded theory is generally considered to lead to the development of categories that will summarise the central elements of the data, but in addition the development of a model that explains how the ideas interrelate. The process of analysis is detailed and systematic and involves intensively scrutinising the data, often sentence by sentence, using constant comparison where the grouping of categories is checked and even rebuilt as the analysis proceeds. The focus of the analysis is not to merely collect and order data but to organise ideas that have emerged from the analysis. Researchers will often refer to emergent theory that develops as ideas are put together, and which itself directs further data collection and analysis. This is because data analysis takes place alongside data collection, which continues until a point known as theoretical saturation, where no new categories emerge and further modification of the theory is trivial. It is important to note that grounded theory allows for modification of the original research question through the process of data collection and analysis.

Of course it could be argued that it is unlikely that any theory can be purely data-derived, since all data interpretation can be influenced by the researcher. Researchers using grounded theory would start with a 'foreshadowed problem' but it has to be acknowledged that being involved in the process of analysis and having personal opinions on the problem being investigated can mean that the researchers themselves affect the formation of the theory. So that even grounded theory, according to some, cannot make the claim to be completely inductive (derived from the data). It is important to acknowledge the impact of the researcher in the research. After all, researchers are part of the social world being studied. Therefore, it is also important for researchers to be reflexive and to discuss how their own experiences/attitudes may have influenced their interpretation and selection of themes as well as the conclusions. In general, grounded theory is considered to be a useful method of analysis that allows researchers to generate 'the truth' from, say, the observation/data itself without the requirement for a pre-existing theory.

Thematic analysis

Thematic analysis is a widely used qualitative analytic method. It involves the analysis of text to generate themes but not necessarily to form a theory. So while thematic analysis is a way of organising qualitative material to draw out meanings, this can be simply in the form of ideas, subject matter and assertions in one person or across different people. Thematic analysis is widely used because it can be related to a variety of theoretical frameworks, such as the social constructionist framework – the view that language is used to construct the way in which one sees the world. In ontological terms, thematic analysis considers that people are able to reflect on their experiences to produce meanings and make sense of them. While researchers using thematic analysis can use the data to derive the themes, similar to grounded theory, themes can then be related back to existing theory in the literature. Thematic analysis can also be theory-driven from the start so that a previous theory is used to lead the research before any analysis begins.

Researchers using thematic analysis will normally work through a series of steps to ultimately produce the overarching themes. The process of coding can involve initially forming descriptive coding, then combining these codes and ultimately generating the general pattern via thematic analysis. The aim is to produce large-scale patterns that draw together the initial codes, ideally accompanied by quotations to exemplify them. Eventually a narrative can be formed to link the themes and summarise the main ideas. Thematic analysis must be seen to be grounded in theory, to be addressing the initial research question and importantly to be rooted in the data analysed.

Discourse analysis

The term discourse analysis covers a number of practices, which generally explore the relationship between communication, understanding, social traditions and power through analysis of language. Discourse analysis takes a strong constructionist position and considers that language is used to create different versions of the truth; it focuses on the way people make meaning and looks at how their 'talk', dialogue, conversation is put together. The epistemological position then is that knowledge is constructed in discourse and the ontological position is that people construct discourse and are constructed by discourse. There are several assumptions upon which discourse analysis is based and these include a belief that people choose how to describe themselves and others; these choices are related to broader social history and are taken for granted because of existing power relations; meanings emerge in social interactions; words and dialogue are a form of social interaction; and finally that words make things real and create identities and positions for people as well as help form memories, intentions and emotions.

A number of concepts are important to discourse analysis including participants' orientations, narrative, voice, interpretative repertoires and subject positions. Briefly, participants' orientation relates to the turn-by-turn nature of conversation, voice relates to the use of others' speech in language, narrative relates to the manner in which people order and give structure to their talk, interpretative repertoires relates to the typical description of things and the broader cultural resources found in talk, and finally subject position relates to the manner in which people construct an identity and a subjectivity for themselves through their narrative. Unlike grounded theory, the aim of discourse analysis is not to produce a complete analysis of all the material in a text or transcript but to analyse the text to uncover, for example, the way in which knowledge and power are created and maintained. One analysis may be different from another. Generally speaking, discourse analysis is conducted by researchers who have developed specific analytical expertise for this purpose.

A note about research ethics

It is important to mention at this stage that there are ethical considerations associated with any research concerning pharmacy practice that is undertaken with human participants. All researchers must be familiar with ethical considerations and they must also demonstrate in their work that they have followed the relevant guidelines. Codes of practice are normally based on moral principles governing research with human participants. Participants must be protected from experiencing psychological or physical harm as a result of taking part in research, and all researchers must maintain moral standards and values, showing respect for participants at all times. The consequences of research are not always predictable and guidelines are in place to ensure researchers think thoroughly through the implications of their research beforehand and any impact the research might have on the participants. Proposals for research will normally have to be reviewed and approved by an ethics committee before being agreed.

Pharmacy practice researchers can be said to have a dual obligation: to advance knowledge and understanding about human interaction and behaviour as it relates to pharmacy in order to benefit society as a whole, and to protect the individuals involved as research participants. The answer to ethical problems is not always clear cut and can involve a cost–benefit analysis. However, it is important to ensure that ethical principles for conducting research with human participants are being followed. Some of these principles include informed consent, participant anonymity, right to withdraw and debriefing, covered briefly below.

Informed consent relates to participants' right to prior knowledge about the nature and the purpose of the research, their agreement to take part in the research based on this understanding but also their right to withdraw at any time and to request that their data are withdrawn from the research. Anonymity relates to participants' right to expect that their identity will not be revealed by either name or any other description. Participants have the right to withdraw from any study at any point of the research without adverse consequences for them and they should be informed at the outset of this right and told also that they may decline to answer particular questions or topics too. In qualitative research in particular, participants have the right to view the findings and interpretations and to withdraw as a result if they so wish. Finally, debriefing of participants involves a mutual discussion between researcher and participant at the end of the study to fully convey the purpose of the research and the likely results and conclusions, to correct any misapprehensions and importantly to ascertain if the participant has experienced any harm or discomfort from the research which necessitates the intervention of a trained specialist.

Conclusion

It should be clear from reading this chapter that much thought will accompany any research project even before it starts. Researchers must not only ensure that they conduct and analyse research appropriately but also protect the research participants throughout the process of research. This chapter has explained differences between two opposing philosophical standpoints and related these to the different methodologies adopted in pharmacy practice research. You should now have at least an understanding of the rationale for conducting different types of research related to pharmaceutical sociology and psychology. Importantly, you are encouraged to apply this understanding of research practices to scrutinise the credibility of social and psychological theory and knowledge generated through research. Indeed this could start with the next four chapters, which outline some of the key psychological and sociological theories relevant to pharmacy through a similar process of description and use of explanatory examples.

Sample examination questions

Students may wish to use the following sample questions to aid their learning and revision before examinations.

1 Define what is meant by research, using examples to illustrate your answer.

2 Describe the fundamentals of grounded theory and thematic analysis.

3 Contrast interpretation with empiricism as two philosophical approaches to research.

4 Summarise salient points in relation to quantitative psychosocial research.

5 Demonstrate the usefulness of qualitative psychosocial research methodology to pharmacy.

6 Justify the importance of quantitative psychosocial research to pharmacy.

7 To what extent does epistemology relate to the type of data generated?

References and further reading

Abercrombi N *et al.* (2000). *The Penguin Dictionary of Sociology*. London: Penguin Group.
Coolican H (2009). *Research Methods and Statistics in Psychology*, 5th edn. London: Hodder Education.

Glaser BG, Strauss AL (1967). *The Discovery of Grounded Theory: Strategies for Qualitative Research*. New York: Aldine de Gruyter.

Yates S (2004). *Doing Social Science Research*. London: Sage Publications.

BMJ Practice series on qualitative research

Hodges BD *et al.* (2008). Discourse analysis. *BMJ*, **337**. doi: 10.1136/bmj.a879.

Kuper A *et al.* (2008). Critically appraising qualitative research. *BMJ*, **337**. doi: 10.1136/bmj.a1035.

Kuper A *et al.* (2008). An introduction to reading and appraising qualitative research. *BMJ*, **337**. doi: 10.1136/bmj.a288.

Lingard L *et al.* (2008). Grounded theory, mixed methods, and action research. *BMJ*, **337**. doi: 10.1136/bmj.39602.690162.47.

Reeves S *et al.* (2008). Why use theories in qualitative research? *BMJ*, **337**. doi: 10.1136/bmj.a949.

Reeves S *et al.* (2008). Qualitative research methodologies: ethnography. *BMJ*, **337**. doi: 10.1136/bmj.a1020.

3

Underpinning psychological theories

Synopsis

Chapter 1 states that psychology is the study of the human mind and its functions as it relates to human cognition, behaviour and experience. The chapter also examines in detail the social determinants of health and disease. It is argued that because a number of behaviours are associated with ill health and behaviour change is seen as a viable way of tackling behaviours associated with health inequalities, pharmacists should therefore be equipped with the tools required to affect their patients' health and illness-related behaviour at the individual level.

This chapter explains human behaviour by exploring psychology in some detail. It presents an overview of a number of underpinning psychological theories relevant to pharmacy practice. The perspective taken is principally that of cognitive psychology – as opposed to, for example, a biological or evolutionary perspective. The key feature of this chapter is that it uses examples to illustrate psychological theories in a pharmacy practice context – something that is developed in Chapters 4 and 5. Another key feature is the arrangement of the chapter into two main parts, with the first providing a basic framework for relating thought to decision making and behaviour, and the second part providing a basic framework for understanding the role of emotion in behaviour.

Learning outcomes

You should be able to demonstrate knowledge and understanding of the following after working through this chapter:

- the relationship between thoughts and the decision-making process
- the interplay of thoughts and emotions.

Introduction

The current chapter focuses on providing the underpinning psychological knowledge. Because decisions can impact on health behaviours, this chapter first examines the mechanism through which thoughts influence decisions. There is then an exploration of emotion and its interrelationship with thought and behaviour. The influence of thought on behaviour and therefore on health can be understood with the help of cognitive psychology, which is a branch of psychology concerned with the operation of the human mind. Social cognition is helpful too, as it links cognition with the social world in situ. Human cognitive processes include perception, attention, memory, learning, thinking, problem solving, decision making and language (Braisby and Gellatly 2005). Although not all of these subjects can be tackled in one chapter, cognitive psychology can be explored for its explanation of information processing in the mind as it relates to decision making.

How can thoughts influence human decisions?

How do people make decisions? Normative theories of decision making centre on ideal decision making – what ought to happen in a perfect model (Thornton *et al.* 1992). Although normative theories attempt to define the perfect decision, they are dependent on a specific view of human rationality, where it is in fact possible to make an 'optimal' decision. Rationality is the ability to use reason to make decisions, for example, regarding possible actions or to determine the optimal choice. But people can also make decisions in the absence of clear information and these decisions can appear irrational to others. In fact, in the real world, people are often faced with information that is either partial or vague, and so decisions are made by what appear to be 'leaps in the dark'. A possible explanation is that, unlike what is suggested by normative theories, people do not operate with machine-like logic, so they resort instead to thought processes that appear to be reasonable to them at the time.

Exploring the concept: decision making in an imperfect situation

For example, imagine being asked to take part in a health questionnaire on your next visit to the supermarket. You might be tempted to take part when you hear that all completed surveys are entered into a prize draw. You imagine that your entry might win you a holiday to Florida. On the other hand, if you stop to complete the survey, you might miss your scheduled bus, which would mean a long walk home in the dark or the rain. What if the confidentiality of the information you provide is breached and your health insurance is affected? What if you win the holiday and meet your future partner in Florida? What are all the pros and cons of completing or indeed not completing the survey and how likely are they to occur? What is the value you attach to each outcome? Normative theories assume it is possible for people to apply this level of analysis when faced with unclear choices and that indeed a perfect decision exists. But how can ideal decision making be possible for humans without the application of a sophisticated algorithm or an exhaustive comparison of all available options? An alternative view is that, under conditions of uncertainty, choices are based on rules-of-thumb. The last time you completed a health questionnaire, it took you too long and you didn't win the prize – decision made. You politely decline and move on.

One justification for this line of thinking is that people build models of the world – schemata – which they then use to understand subsequent social interactions (Miell *et al.* 2007). From a biological perspective it is thought that humans need to keep cognitive processes minimal to make the best use of the processing capacity in the brain, which has resulted in the formation of schema theory. People's schemata are their own generalised representations of social phenomena based on shared knowledge about people/events/roles/objects as stereotypes. A schema about something (e.g., a type of profession) helps people recognise and understand it better the next time they encounter an example of it (building a picture of a physiotherapist in the mind, including what to expect can help in later interactions with the same or indeed other physiotherapists). You might think of this process as stereotyping. Another helpful concept here is that of heuristics, which relates in particular to judgement and decision making when knowledge is vague (Gigerenzer and Gaissmaier 2011). Heuristics are strategies based on readily available mental representations of the world, which can be evoked during decision making to make the process more efficient. It is thought that people's access to heuristics helps them make decisions under uncertainty. This approach is in contrast to normative theories, which, as briefly outlined above, are based on the attainability of the perfect choice.

The idea of heuristics relies on a more pragmatic view of rationality, which is that cognitive processes are not designed to return rational decisions so cannot be guaranteed to ever produce 'optimal' outcomes. This view of cognition is known as 'bounded rationality' – the notion that in truth human rationality is limited by the mind's ability to completely process all the information necessary to arrive at the perfect 'rational' choice (Chase *et al.* 1998).

Since thorough and exhaustive scrutiny of all available information is not normally achievable, the concept of bounded rationality necessitates the use of alternative systems, for example, heuristics, to arrive at decisions. Heuristics draw on people's propensity to access readily available mental representations, for example, rules-of-thumb or schemata, to inform their choices. The idea of heuristics enables rationality to operate outside of normative theories, to fall in line with real-life experiences.

A brief examination of heuristics

An array of heuristics has been investigated and proposed (Braisby and Gellatly 2005). Psychologists investigating people's decision making under conditions of uncertainty have identified, for example:

- the anchoring and adjustment heuristic
- the availability heuristic
- the representativeness heuristic.

Anchoring and adjustment heuristic

The anchoring and adjustment heuristic operates when people estimate the answer to a question based on an initial value presented to them as part of the question.

Exploring the concept: the anchoring and adjustment heuristic

Imagine the supermarket example again but this time in the context of the pharmacy counter. In fact, you are the locum pharmacist and today, a Saturday, is your first day at the store. On signing the responsible pharmacist register, the technician makes a comment about the number of pharmacists who locum at the store. She asks if you can guess whether this number is higher or lower than 20. You make an estimate and guess 17. What if the technician had asked whether you think the number is higher or lower than 5? According to the anchoring and adjustment heuristic, the initial value posed in such a question (the anchor) acts as a basis for the answer, albeit it is adjusted to some extent to yield the final estimate.

Availability heuristic

The availability heuristic operates when people predict the likelihood of something by the ease with which similar instances can be recalled.

Exploring the concept: the availability heuristic

Now imagine you are halfway through the same locum-day and a patient asks you for the best over-the-counter product for a chesty cough. The (fictional) brand Best-for-Cough comes to mind. The recent television advertisement claimed this product is effective in 95% of cases. You immediately reach for Best-for-Cough's new Chesty Mucus Cough formulation. Is the product more likely to work compared with any other product or are you making the recommendation because the words in the advert come to mind? According to the availability heuristic the frequency or probability of an event (e.g., the probability of the product being effective) is judged by the number of instances of it that can easily be brought to mind. Other products may be just as effective but if they are not 'on the radar' so to speak, they are less likely to be recommended.

Representativeness heuristic

The representativeness heuristic is used when people categorise things/events by considering their similarity to the group/category.

Exploring the concept: the representativeness heuristic

Finally, and again in the same scenario, imagine being told in advance that although hectic, Saturdays provide one relief because the two very difficult customers who are sisters and can be identified by their characteristic beret and cape, and who insist on buying multiple packs of codeine, normally only visit during the week. Then imagine an elderly lady approaches the pharmacy counter near closing time to ask for a strong painkiller, preferably containing codeine. You might well think that this lady is one of the 'difficult' sisters you were warned about earlier because she fits the general perceived characteristics. According to the representative heuristic people estimate the probability that an item belongs to a category by judging the degree to which the item is representative or typical of the category.

A brief examination of cognitive biases

The human propensity to use heuristics, although helpful, can also lead to erroneous judgements because of a concept known as cognitive bias, the by-product of making decisions under bounded rationality (Tversky and Kahneman 1974). For example, mainly through experimental research, heuristics have been linked to the following biases, which have been recognised in medical practice – for example, see Klein (2005) and Bornstein and Emler (2001) (Fig. 3.1):

- the overconfidence bias
- the base-rate fallacy
- the conjunction fallacy
- the sample size fallacy
- the regression fallacy
- the framing effect.

Using the experimental method to study social cognition must of course be treated with some degree of caution, as studying phenomena (which are social) in the laboratory rather than in situ can lead to questions of ecological validity – with the potential that results produced in the laboratory are not exact reflections of the social *truth*. After all, people in the laboratory are not faced with any sense of real urgency and are not connected emotionally with the experimental scenarios, as they would normally be in the outside world. Nonetheless, where a positivist epistemology is subscribed to and questions are framed appropriately, the experimental method does enable social phenomena to be studied in a less complex and more controlled manner.

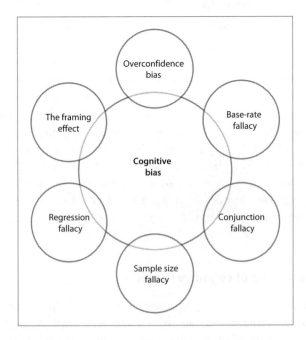

Figure 3.1 Examples of different types of cognitive bias associated with the use of heuristics.

Overconfidence bias

Now returning to the different types of erroneous judgements, the overconfidence bias concerns claims that people's expressions of confidence in the accuracy of their own judgements are largely unreliable, resulting in higher confidence ratings when measured against actual correctness.

Exploring the concept: the overconfidence bias

Let's return to the supermarket pharmacy where you are a locum on that Saturday. Imagine being asked by a patient whether it is paracetamol or ibuprofen that is safer in early pregnancy. What about aspirin versus ibuprofen or paracetamol versus aspirin? How confident would you be of the accuracy of your judgement each time? The overconfidence bias concerns claims that people's expressions of confidence in the accuracy of their own judgements are largely unreliable, resulting in overconfidence when measured against correctness. What are the consequences of the overconfidence bias for patients involved in self-care, for example?

Base-rate fallacy

The base-rate fallacy is the failure to take account of the prior probability of an event when making a judgement.

Exploring the concept: the base-rate fallacy

Remember the thinking, again in a previous example, that the elderly patient approaching the counter was one of the 'difficult' sisters, despite the fact that staff had explained the sisters only normally visited during the week (the baseline probability of a visit was low). A base-rate fallacy could have occurred, as a result of the failure to take in the actual probability of a visit by the sisters when making the judgement.

Conjunction fallacy

The conjunction fallacy is an error according to which a combination of two or more attributes is judged more probable than either attribute on its own.

Exploring the concept: the conjunction fallacy

Now supposing a patient came into the pharmacy expressing concern that based on her symptoms and information on the internet she fears a diagnosis of ulcerative colitis. She has read about treatment options and also fears that if the doctor makes this diagnosis and prescribes her the relevant medication, she will experience the severe side-effects she has read about. In fact, she strongly believes that if she visits the doctor she is more likely to end up with an exacerbation of her symptoms due to side-effects of medication than just be diagnosed with ulcerative colitis. This is a fallacy because the concurrence of being diagnosed with ulcerative colitis and finding herself with worse symptoms caused by the medication cannot exceed the probability of the diagnosis alone. The conjunction fallacy is an error according to which a combination of two or more attributes is judged more probable than either attribute on its own.

Sample-size fallacy

The sample-size fallacy is also important. It describes the failure to take account of the sample size when estimating the probability of obtaining a particular value in a sample obtained from a particular population.

Exploring the concept: the sample-size fallacy

Imagine in this same scenario that normally around 300 patients visit the pharmacy every day to purchase an over-the-counter product from the healthcare assistant. What is the likelihood that an unusually high number of patients will ask to consult with you, the pharmacist, in any one day? What would be the likelihood if you worked there for a week or a month or a year? You might think the probability is the same in all cases but in actual fact the probability of an unusually high sample average is much greater in a small sample (one day) than in a larger one (one month) – think of the normal distribution. The sample-size fallacy is a failure to take account of sample size when estimating the probability of a particular rate in a sample taken from a larger population. This erroneous pattern of belief is explained by the use of the representativeness heuristic, which is not sensitive to sample size. A common form of the sample-size fallacy is people's inclination to think that a small sample is typical of its parent population.

Regression fallacy

The regression fallacy is a mistaken assumption that interprets regression towards the mean as attributable to something other than chance.

Exploring the concept: the regression fallacy

Now suppose a particular patient does ask to see you, and interestingly, with a theory about her visits to the pharmacy. On speaking with her, you discover she has formed a particular belief relating to her experience of the pharmacy, which does not quite ring true. The patient explains that when she visits the pharmacy during the week, the pharmacist sometimes makes extra time to speak with her and so the patient leaves feeling very 'looked after' and content. Yet if the patient has a particularly good interaction with the pharmacy one day, when she returns the next time, she somehow ends up leaving the premises less satisfied. Curiously, the next visit after that will usually lead to a better interaction again and so on. In fact, the patient has come to believe that a good interaction is somehow counterproductive to her future experiences of the pharmacy and that a colder interaction is in some way better overall. In reality, because of a regression towards the mean, good or bad experiences are just as likely to be followed by an average one, which explains the resultant feeling. The regression fallacy is a mistaken assumption that interprets natural regression towards the mean as attributable to something other than chance.

Framing effect

Finally, the framing effect describes the impact that the explanation, labelling or arrangement of a problem can have on responses to the problem. This is particularly important in pharmacy, where patient information leaflets attempt to convey medication-related facts in product packaging, and where advertising is used to convey effectiveness data for medicines on the market.

Exploring the concept: the framing effect

A final example using the locum pharmacy scenario, involves an interesting interaction with a patient who brings in a cutting from a well-known national tabloid. The cutting is in fact an advert for a new 'miracle cure' for arthritis, claiming it to be 33% better compared with prescription-only anti-inflammatory medication. On closer examination you note the advert in fact relates to the purported safety of the herb *Boswellia*. The small print reports the outcome of a small study where 15 of 100 patients taking non-steroidal anti-inflammatory drugs (NSAIDs) reported stomach problems compared with only 10 of 100 patients taking *Boswellia*. Taking these numbers at face value, the 33% relates to the relative risk reduction in reported stomach pains. Using the same data, the absolute risk reduction in stomach pains would be expressed as 5%. This is not as impressive and yet the patient is clearly impressed with *Boswellia*. Is it likely that the absolute risk reduction figure would have been used in the advert? Would your patient's response have been the same? The framing effect describes the impact that the explanation, labelling or arrangement of a problem can have on responses to the problem.

What is attribution theory?

An interesting and related concept concerns the interplay between schemata and motivation in the form of attribution theory. The psychologist Fritz Heider believed that people use schemata to build models of the world, which they then use to understand *why other people do what they do* – this particular idea is known as 'attribution theory' (Braisby and Gellatly 2005). Attribution theory can help us understand the way in which people perceive and explain their social environment, specifically in relation to the reasons they give for other people's behaviour in the form of feelings, beliefs and intentions. Although it may appear from the discussions earlier in the chapter that schemata effectively dominate people's thinking, Ruscher *et al.* (as cited in Buchanan *et al.* 2007), through carefully planned experiments, showed that *motivation* can also play a role when considering, in particular, people's decisions about others. So, for example, a simple conceptualisation of schema theory might be too reductionist and as such not take account of the human capacity to think outside of the confines of their biology. Fiske and Taylor (as cited in Buchanan *et al.* 2007) suggested people act as 'motivated tacticians' and 'fully engaged thinkers who have multiple cognitive strategies available and choose among them based on goals, motives and needs'.

Theories of attribution have been developed to understand the reasons behind ours and others' actions. The experimental method has been used extensively in relation to attribution theory and related research – to develop generalisable theories about the social world. One of the earlier experiments used by Heider and Simmel (as cited in Buchanan *et al.* 2007) provides convincing evidence that people form narratives to match their observation of others and events. In terms of understanding other people's behaviour, Heider argued that people ascribe internal or external causes to others' behaviour, along a continuum of causality. Jones and Davis (as cited in Buchanan *et al.* 2007) contributed to this work by suggesting that people tend to ascribe internal causes to others' behaviour more than to their own, in an attempt perhaps to understand the person rather than merely their action.

Exploring the concept: attribution theory

Imagine receiving the wrong medication from your own local pharmacist. What would be your reaction in terms of apportioning blame? Would you think the pharmacist a careless and sloppy worker or might you blame their employer for not providing sufficient staff to help with second-checking of dispensed items? A comment relating to the pharmacist's character, as a sloppy worker, for example, is an internal attribution of blame (there is something internal within the pharmacist that has resulted in the accident) whereas blaming the working conditions is an external attribution.

Harold Kelley went so far as to devise a *co-variation matrix* suggesting that, in struggling to make sense of other people's actions and in wanting to assign the cause of specific behaviour as internal or external, people fit knowledge of others' past actions to current situations in a systematic manner using three variables of consistency, distinctiveness and consensus. This structured approach has enabled scientific verification of Kelley's theory through experimental methods, for example, through the use of vignettes that offer selective information, based on which participants form causality judgements (as cited in Buchanan *et al.* 2007). Using vignettes is an example of an experimental method with potentially low ecological validity, since reduction of events to much controlled levels can mean detachment from real, everyday experiences.

Exploring the concept: Kelley's co-variation matrix

Kelley believed people combine three types of information to explain behaviour: consensus, consistency and distinctiveness. Imagine coming into work one Monday to find one of your technicians smelling of alcohol, acting out of character and upsetting the healthcare assistants. In relation to this behaviour, consensus is the behaviour's similarity to other people's behaviour – how unusual is this behaviour in general? In the context of pharmacy, it would be fair to say it's unusual to find technicians arriving at work drunk on a Monday morning! However, is drinking to excess particularly unusual? Consensus might therefore be judged as high (this behaviour is perhaps not that unusual for the general UK population?) Consistency is the degree to which this particular event is similar to the person's past behaviour in a similar situation – is this typical behaviour for the technician on a Monday morning? From the above information, it does not seem that this is the technician's typical behaviour at work. Consistency is therefore also low (not typical of the technician in this situation). Distinctiveness is the extent to which the behaviour is uncharacteristic in general. Does the technician normally drink excessively, say outside of work? Imagine the technician normally abstains from drink. Distinctiveness is therefore high (this is not something the technician does in other circumstances). According to Kelley, people attribute others' behaviour to external, situational causes when consensus is high, consistency low and distinctiveness high – such as in this example – whereas they attribute internal causes when consensus is low, consistency is high, and distinctiveness is low.

Critics have pointed out with some evidence that Kelley's theory overstates the rationality of people's reasoning, perhaps because the experimental method cannot take into account the complexity of social life. For example, in everyday situations, as alluded to above, people explain the behaviour of others using internal attributions, a tendency known as *fundamental attribution error* – whereas they tend to select external attributions for explaining their own behaviour (known as the *actor/observer effect*). But fundamental attribution error may not have universal application. Miller (as cited in Buchanan *et al.* 2007) has shown through experiments using American participants versus Indian Hindu participants that culture and ideology may underlie attributional preferences. Western culture is more individualistic than many cultures in the East and may be impacting on people's attention when attributing cause, and thus causing fundamental attribution error. (Attributing internal causes to others' behaviour may just be unique in the West, where the culture is more individualistic.)

Exploring the concept: fundamental attribution error and the actor/observer effect

We will return here to the dispensing error example, above. According to fundamental attribution error, you (the patient) would be much more likely to blame the pharmacist for the dispensing error, a flaw in their character or style of working perhaps, than any external factors. According to the actor/observer effect, however, the pharmacist is much more likely to blame something external to themselves for the error, such as the working conditions or a sudden rush of patients.

Another aspect of attribution research that helps us understand the way in which people perceive and explain their social environment is related to the *self-serving bias* of causal attribution, where successes are related to internal causes and failures to external ones. Self-serving bias has in fact been linked to cognitive bias – where attributions are based on thought processes, such as those relating to expectations rather than objective facts. Another way in which self-serving bias has been explained is through motivational bias linked to a need to present explanations in the best possible light, perhaps to boost self-esteem. There are difficulties with such theories though. For example, while Shrauger (as cited in Buchanan *et al.* 2007) found that those with higher self-esteem tended to make more self-serving attributions than those with low self-esteem, the direction of causation is unclear since either high self-esteem or self-serving attributions could be the cause or the effect. Nonetheless, there is evidence that attribution can impact on people's sense of self.

Exploring the concept: the self-serving bias

Imagine you are a hospital pharmacist in charge of medicines information services. An overhaul of your department means queries are now dealt with more efficiently than before. A review of the services returns an excellent rating. According to the self-serving bias, you are much more likely to attribute this 'success' to your and your team's hard work than any external factors (and why not!). On the other hand, imagine that the overhaul means queries take longer to deal with and the review returns a poor rating. According to the self-serving bias, you are much more likely to blame external factors for this rating than yourself – for example, you might make a case that the number of queries has unexpectedly increased in the period since the overhaul, or that budget cuts have lowered the total human resource available to answer the queries.

Human decision making can be error-prone, and research investigating people's performance on making formal judgements can suggest that humans are fundamentally irrational in their decision making. Yet there is also compelling evidence that humans do manage to live and operate in an uncertain world alongside one another. Indeed in real life, decisions are made using 'fast and frugal heuristics', simplified and speedy processing of information under bounded rationality (Gigerenzer and Gaissmaier 2011). Here, human decision making has been found to be highly accurate so it is important to consider heuristics and biases in the context in which they are naturally used, rather than contrived experimental settings. One natural setting of course relates to decision making in relation to health, which is the focus of Chapter 4. Here, building on this basic overview of thought and decision making, the interplay of emotion and thought is examined next.

What is the interrelationship between emotions and thoughts?

An exploration of emotion and its impact on thought and behaviour warrants particular consideration in the context of ill health, as does the converse relationship, which is the effect of thoughts and behaviour on emotion. Thus, before examining models that relate specifically to people's experiences of health and disease management in Chapters 4 and 5, the mechanisms through which emotion and thought interrelate will be examined. A typical view is that the concept of emotion is different from that of cognition – cognition is concerned with knowledge acquisition whereas emotion relates to feelings and mood. In addition, the field of psychology has traditionally focused to a greater extent on studying and defining cognitive processes than it has on emotion. However, research on emotion and specifically the interplay between cognition and emotion is also important, especially in relation to ill health where it is not uncommon for people to experience an initial or ongoing emotional response to their condition. How someone feels can influence their thoughts but interestingly how they think can also affect their feelings, and so on, but how closely linked are these two concepts?

Emotion relates to feelings and mood, which can be conceptualised in a number of ways (Izard 2009). The experience of emotion can be related to three components: subjectively experienced feelings, expression of emotion via a behavioural response, and a physiological response to emotion (Fig. 3.2). For example, fear of visiting the doctor can involve an unpleasant subjective experience of dread, a behavioural response that drives the person away from the doctor's practice, and a measurable physiological response such as increased blood pressure. The different types of emotion can be conceptualised in terms of basic emotions, such as the five emotions of anger, fear, sadness, disgust and happiness, or in a more sophisticated dimensional manner, as an interaction between emotion-related valence (pleasant/unpleasant) with arousal (calm/aroused). Evolutionary psychologists have even proposed a role for emotion in goal attainment, in mobilising physiological resources and in communication, and emotion is even considered by some as a source of information (Braisby and Gellatly 2005).

Can emotion influence thought and behaviour and vice versa?

Psychologists have been able to study and demonstrate with strong and varied evidence that emotion can affect thought. Experiments have been used to demonstrate the impact of (the processing of) emotion on different cognitive processes including memory, attention and semantic interpretation (construal of meaning) (Braisby and Gellatly 2005) (Fig. 3.3). Briefly, emotion can affect memory by influencing the coding of memory and indeed the recall of memory. In fact it has been found that clinically depressed patients, or

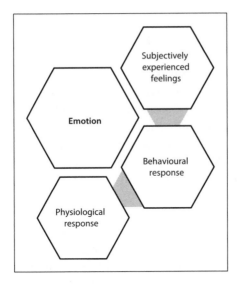

Figure 3.2 Conceptualising the experience of emotion. (Data from Izard 2009.)

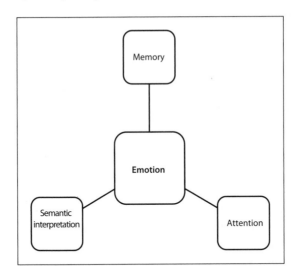

Figure 3.3 Conceptualising the effect of emotion on thought processes. (Data from Braisby and Gellatly 2005.)

those in constantly low mood, all show a negative 'bias' in terms of coding memory (i.e., are more likely to code negative material), despite the fact that 'normal' individuals have a positive (rather than neutral) bias towards memory. It has been suggested that the bias itself acts to reinforce depression in a vicious cycle. Indeed, such theories have formed the basis of interventions that attempt to break the cycle and thus alter cognition in order to *impact on emotion*.

Exploring the concept: the impact of emotion on memory

Imagine you are experiencing a period of work-related stress because your department is under-resourced. Then you become involved in an altercation with one of the clinical pharmacists about the ward rota. Your colleague suggests that while you have carried out thorough and careful wards visit that morning, you have neglected to cover all the wards assigned to you. You become annoyed at the insinuation that you have somehow neglected to do your job properly and begin to recall other instances of what you consider to be 'harassment' by the same colleague. On later describing the event, you recount a very negative interpretation of the disagreement, neglecting to recall any of the positive comments your colleague made about your work ethos. The distressed frame of mind during the argument meant that not only did you recall other instances of unconstructive events but your mind also worked to embed to memory only the negative elements of the interaction. What impact might the relationship between mood and memory have on the way distressed patients deal with information about their illness?

In addition to memory, the effect of emotion on attention, another aspect of cognition, has also been studied through experimental research. There is evidence of an *anxiety-related attentional bias* in certain individuals (i.e., in those who have an anxious trait, and indeed in clinically anxious patients such as those with post-traumatic stress disorder) (Braisby and Gellatly 2005). This means that anxious individuals are more likely to pay attention (depending on the experimental design) to emotional, negative or threatening words. Therefore, here researchers have suggested the existence of another vicious cycle in real life similar to that described above, where the emotion-induced *cognitive bias* then actually further impacts on emotion, reinforcing, in this example, the anxiety of the individual. Indeed, there have been some experimental attempts to reverse the effect of this bias, with some success.

Exploring the concept: the impact of emotion on attention

Imagine a patient diagnosed with type 2 diabetes, who has not been coping at all well with their diagnosis and disease management. The pharmacist conducts a Medicines Use Review, making sure to explain the continuing need for regular eye checks, foot care and blood pressure measurements as well as ensuring a healthy diet. The pharmacist follows his normal style and attempts to reinforce his message by explaining the consequences of failing to act in accordance with his advice. If the patient is already worried, they may focus more on the negative effects of diabetes, as emphasised by the pharmacist, than on the more positive words relating to prevention or postponement of these effects. This could further affect the patient's emotional state.

The final cognitive process thought to be influenced by emotion and considered here, is that of semantic interpretation of meaning (Braisby and Gellatly 2005). Again, through experimentation, researchers have unearthed an emotional impact on cognition, in the form of an interpretative bias, where, for example, participants who are anxious might be more likely to form a negative interpretation of words that have multiple meanings. Conversely, non-anxious participants display a positive bias, leading to the concept of protective processing styles such as attribution theory and the self-serving attribution bias. Here one could argue that the existence of the positive bias has a role in helping maintain good mood and a positive self-image.

Exploring the concept: the impact of emotion on semantic interpretation

Imagine a distressed patient overhearing a dispensary conversation. The pharmacist is talking with their pre-registration trainee about red, sugar-coated tablets. The trainee mentions excipients and red dye and the pharmacist repeats 'Yes, that's a good point, definitely dye'. According to the theory linking emotion to semantic interpretation, the patient might be more likely to attach negative meanings to words with multiple meanings, if they are anxious at the time. On hearing this excerpt, the patient might hear *die* instead of *dye*.

The above examples all focus on the impact of *cognition on emotion* as an indirect and iterative consequence of bias that results from the effect of *emotion on cognition* in the social context. That is, a patient making a negative interpretation through their thought processes can experience a further negative effect on their emotion – the negative interpretation itself arising from a negative emotional state due to illness. A separate argument relates to a more fundamental question of whether or not cognition (thought) is necessary before an emotional response is ever elicited.

Three main theories are summarised – for a recent review see Friedman (2010). First, the James–Lange theory (William James and Carl Lange) argues that emotion is a response to stimulus (i.e., behaviour precedes conscious cognition, leading to emotion), while second, the Cannon–Bard theory (Walter Cannon and Philip Bard) argues that autonomic arousal can occur in parallel to the experience of the emotion. Central to the James–Lange theory is the concept that emotion depends on the bodily reaction that follows an event, meaning different physiological signatures are required to produce different feelings. Indeed, there is some evidence to support this idea from patients with spinal injury who are unable to experience physiological changes and emotions despite the presence of emotional stimuli. Yet, Cannon and Bard were also able to provide support for their theory by citing that those with damaged spinal cords where a physiological response to stimuli is prevented, could still respond emotionally (Braisby and Gellatly 2005).

Exploring the concept: the James–Lange theory and the Cannon–Bard theory

Applying the James–Lange theory to a pharmacy situation, we might say that a patient is feeling sorry because they have just cried – or indeed that a pharmacist faced with a threatening client is scared because they have just trembled. Conversely, according to the Cannon–Bard theory, the bodily expression of the patient's emotion (crying), governed by signals from the brain to the muscles and glands, occurs at the same time that the emotion (sadness) is felt.

A third view that contrasts both models above relates to that of Stanley Schachter and Jerome Singer, who proposed a crucial role for the cognitive appraisal of stimuli *before* the experience of emotion takes place. Schachter–Singer thus introduced the concept that cognition can control emotion. For example, they were able to demonstrate that although injecting participants with adrenaline can lead to the experience of emotion, the emotional response could also be controlled by individuals through cognitive processes and also that the experience of emotion was strongly linked to the social and physical experience of study participants. Other appraisal theorists have since shared this notion, that emotions are experienced as they are because of individual assessment of the stimuli, yet theorists have tended to suggest different sets of dimensions used by people when making such appraisals (Braisby and Gellatly 2005). For example, there are the Schachter appraisal criteria.

Exploring the concept: the Schachter–Singer theory

Imagine you are away and staying on the fifth floor of an old hotel in a room at the far end of the corridor. Exactly at midnight, you are woken up by the loud siren of the hotel's fire alarm. You will undoubtedly experience a range of emotions such as fear and anger as you try to leave your room. On the other hand, imagine the same experience. This time you have the prior knowledge that owing to a fault in the hotel's system, you should expect to hear the sound of the fire bell at exactly midnight. In fact, because of the anticipated inconvenience, your night's stay is half the normal price. With this prior knowledge, is it likely that you would experience the same range of emotions on being woken up at midnight? According to the Schachter–Singer theory, cognitive appraisal of stimuli takes place before emotion is experienced. That is, a person's interpretation (cognitive evaluation) plays a key role in determining the ensuing emotion.

Historically, Richard Lazarus, whose theories will also be discussed in Chapter 5, was a proponent of appraisal theory, and was strongly challenged by Robert Zajonc – who in turn did not believe that appraisal was a necessary precursor of emotion, sparking a debate about whether cognition precedes emotion or *vice versa*, referred to as the primacy debate (Braisby and Gellatly 2005). Although Lazarus and Zajonc were able to provide some experimental evidence in support of their individual positions on this, more recently Joseph LeDoux (cited in Braisby and Gellatly 2005) has demonstrated that both positions may be valid. LeDoux has suggested the existence of two alternative pathways in the brain taking information from the point where stimuli are perceived to where the emotional response is elicited. The first, a primitive 'lower' route, bypasses the higher brain structure and takes information from the sensory thalamus region to the amygdala via one synapse to elicit a fast emotional response; the second, a 'higher' more evolved route, while also taking the information from the thalamus to the amygdala, does this via the sensory cortex. The lower route maps on to Zajonc's ideas, whereas the higher route maps on to ideas put forward by Lazarus, enabling the moderation of emotional response via more sophisticated cognitive processes involving thought and appraisal.

Proposals relating to cognitive processes that could be used by individuals to *regulate emotional responses* also warrant brief discussion. For example, Gross and colleagues (cited in Braisby and Gellatly 2005) have contrasted *behavioural* and *cognitive* regulation, the former relating to the suppression of expressive behaviour and the latter to whether the stimulus can be attended to or interpreted in a manner that limits emotional response.

One concept relating to the cognitive regulation of emotion proposes a hypothetical continuum that has at one end attentional control and at another cognitive change (Ochsner and Gross 2005). Attentional control has examined evidence that paying less attention to stimuli can change processing in the amygdala, for example, to influence the emotional appraisal system. Here, both selective attention, focusing on a particular feature of the stimuli, and attentional distraction, limiting attention to emotional stimuli, have been studied. Evidence for attentional control of emotion does exist but it has not shed light on the exact mechanisms and context governing this regulatory effect.

Exploring the concept: the attentional control of emotion

Imagine a patient finds an unusual mole on their skin that appears to be getting larger, potentially indicating early signs of a melanoma. They visit their GP, who refers them to a specialist but that appointment is not for another two days. This delay upsets the patient enormously and they find themselves getting more and more anxious during the wait. If the patient could somehow pay less attention to their mole, would the ensuing two days would be easier to bear? Attentional control has examined evidence that paying less attention to stimuli can influence the emotional appraisal system.

In relation to cognitive change, researchers have begun asking how cognitive abilities can be 'used to construct expectations for, select alternative interpretations of, and/or make different judgements about emotional stimuli that can change both behavioural and neural responses to them' (Ochsner and Gross 2005). Controlled generation and controlled regulation have been examined in this context, with the latter related to cognitive change in the context of an existing or ongoing emotional response. Findings from studies examining cognitive change produce more consistent results (compared with attentional control) which has been attributed to the use of stimuli that produce strong emotional responses as well as regulatory strategies that engage regulatory processes in a clear strong manner.

Exploring the concept: the cognitive control of emotion

Imagine again the same patient as above, with the problematic mole. What is the negative interpretation that is leading to the patient's emotional reaction and what other plausible explanations are there? The discovery of an unusual mole does not equal a terminal prognosis.

What if the patient could be taught to make a different, more balanced interpretation of their symptoms?

It becomes apparent from reviewing the available evidence, not only that cognition and emotion are interlinked, but also that there is a scientific basis for using cognitive and behavioural strategies to influence emotion. This provides a basis for understanding some of the behaviour-change models such as cognitive behaviour therapy, now recommended by the UK health service for dealing with negative interpretations of illness and disease. In fact, in this book cognitive techniques are referred to in the context of better communication in Chapter 6.

Conclusion

People's thoughts and decision making can depend on their ideas about the world and even their emotional state. The way that people think about the world can help them make more efficient decisions or it can hinder the decisional outcome through erroneous thinking. Sometimes people are motivated to think about matters in a way that preserves their sense of self. This could be particularly important in the context of health, where people's emotions will be embroiled in their thought processes. People's emotional state can affect their memory, attention and construction of meaning, impacting in turn on their decision making. Thoughts too can influence people's emotions, with people making an assessment about an event before forming an emotional response. This provides the basis for teaching people the skills to direct their thoughts in more productive ways. While this chapter has examined some fundamental concepts relating to thought and decision making, the next chapter examines health beliefs and behaviour-change models in relation to health (or health-damaging) behaviours.

Sample examination questions

Students may wish to use the following sample questions to aid their learning and revision before examinations:

1   Describe the availability and the representativeness heuristics, using examples to illustrate your answer.

2   Give a definition of cognitive bias associated with the use of heuristics, describing three types of bias in your answer.

3   Summarise your understanding of attribution theory.

4 Justify the importance of the emotion–cognition relationship.

5 Contrast normative ideas with heuristics-based ideas in relation to decision making.

6 To what extent can emotion affect thought processes?

7 Defend the idea that thought can be used to control emotion.

References and further reading

Bornstein BH, Emler AC (2001). Rationality in medical decision making: a review of the literature on doctors' decision-making biases. *Journal of Evaluation in Clinical Practice*, 7: 97–107.

Braisby N, Gellatly A (2005). *Cognitive Psychology*. Oxford: Oxford University Press.

Buchanan K *et al.* (2007). Perceiving and understanding the social world. In: Miell D *et al.*, eds. *Mapping Psychology*. Milton Keynes: The Open University, 57–104.

Chase VM *et al.* (1998). Visions of rationality. *Trends in Cognitive Sciences*, 2: 206–214.

Friedman BH (2010). Feelings and the body: the Jamesian perspective on autonomic specificity of emotion. *Biological Psychology*, **84**: 383–393.

Gigerenzer G, Gaissmaier W (2011). Heuristic decision making. *Annual Review of Psychology*, **62**: 451–482.

Izard CE (2009). Emotion theory and research: highlights, unanswered questions, and emerging issues. *Annual Review of Psychology*, **60**: 1–25.

Klein JG (2005). Five pitfalls in decisions about diagnosis and prescribing. *BMJ*, **330**: 781–784.

Miell D *et al.* (2007). *Mapping Psychology*. Milton Keynes: The Open University.

Ochsner KN, Gross JJ (2005). The cognitive control of emotion. *Trends in Cognitive Sciences*, **9**: 242–249.

Thornton JG *et al.* (1992). Decision analysis in medicine. *BMJ*, **304**: 1099–1103.

Tversky A, Kahneman D (1974). Judgment under uncertainty: heuristics and biases. *Science*, **185**: 1124–1131.

4

Psychological models of health behaviour and behaviour change

Synopsis

Chapter 3 outlined general mechanisms through which thoughts can impact on decision making, and a framework for understanding the interplay between thought and emotion was also examined. It was concluded that the way people think about the world can help them make more efficient decisions or it can hinder the decisional outcome. This chapter explores those concepts further by relating them to people's health behaviours (or health-damaging behaviours). Chapter 4 examines a number of models of health behaviour and their usefulness as evidenced by research. The models are considered in the context of their underlying theoretical bases for bringing about behavioural change, resulting in an assessment of the particular value of each model.

Learning outcomes

You should be able to demonstrate knowledge and understanding of the following after working through this chapter:

- the basis of the *health belief model*, and *social cognitive theory* for explaining behaviour
- the basis, usefulness and limitations of the *integrative model of behavioural prediction* for changing health behaviour
- the basis, usefulness and limitations of the *transtheoretical model* for changing health behaviour
- the basis, usefulness and limitations of the *fuzzy-trace theory* for changing health behaviour.

Introduction

Recall – a number of health-damaging behaviours were discussed in Chapter 1, including smoking, being obese, and alcohol misuse. Numerous specific theories and models offer to explain the link between thoughts, decision making and *risky* (health-damaging) as well as *healthy* behaviours. For example, there is the health belief model, social cognitive theory, the transtheoretical/stage of change model, the theory of planned behaviour, the precede–proceed model, expected utility theory, illness script theory, prospect theory, query theory, social network/social support theory and the counselling-based method of motivational interviewing. Although an array of theories and models attempt to explain the link between thoughts, beliefs, decisions and behaviours, not all theories are helpful or indeed evidence-based, so it is neither essential, nor desirable, to simply study all of these theories.

In addition, it is important to appreciate that although theories might be well-supported by research and in fact 'proven' to work within an experimental setting, not all interventions are practical enough to be of benefit in natural settings. Can people's health-related behaviours ever be predicted and changed? Reviews identify the following theories/cognitive models as having been most used in published research: the transtheoretical model/stages of change, social cognitive theory, health belief model, theory of reasoned action and the theory of planned behaviour. The basis for examining these models is to provide pharmacy professionals with an understanding of theory-based interventions that attempt to help people change their behaviours from health-damaging ones to healthy ones.

Here, first the health belief model and then the social cognitive theory are considered. Then three further examples, the integrative model of behavioural prediction (which combines theory of reasoned action/theory of planned behaviour), the transtheoretical model (also known as stages of change) and fuzzy-trace theory are outlined with particular reference to their rationale and evidence of usefulness. Fuzzy-trace theory has been chosen as a relatively newer theory, which, instead of being founded fully on normative theory, has leanings towards the concept of heuristics and biases outlined in Chapter 3. In explaining the latter three theories, this section draws on the writing of each of the three theories' founders published in a series of papers in the journal *Medical Decision Making*.

Health belief model

The health belief model (HBM) is considered first as it is one of the original theories developed in relation to health behaviours and is still widely referred to in health psychology. Although initial ideas relating to the model originated in the 1950s, Irwin M Rosenstock and Marshall H Becker are often associated with the refinement of the HBM from the 1960s onwards. The HBM is derived from two psychological theories about learning, *stimulus response* and *cognitive theory* (Rosenstock *et al.* 1988), which are considered here briefly, for completion.

Stimulus response, which has its roots in behaviourism, asserts that learning occurs as a result of events. According to this theory then, people learn to avoid behaviour that leads to punishment because they want to avoid the negative experience of being punished – by contrast, the simple association with a reward will increase the chances of repeating a rewarded behaviour. So, in summary, according to stimulus response, behaviour is determined by its consequences – a somewhat simplistic consideration that discounts the influence of more sophisticated cognitive concepts such as thinking and reasoning.

By contrast, cognitive theory emphasises the role of subjective theories, beliefs and expectations held by the individual. Behaviour then becomes a function of the subjective 'value' of an outcome and the subjective 'probability' (expectation) that such an outcome will be achieved as a result of some action or behaviour – a value–expectancy theory. The consequences of a behaviour fit into this type of model by influencing expectations.

The HBM was developed mainly as an explanatory model of why people behave in the way that they do. The underlying assumption of the HBM is that the balance of people's beliefs about the risks associated with a disease or health problem and their perception of the benefits of taking preventative action, will determine their readiness to adopt the desired behaviour (which might avert the disease or health problem). The model has been used widely in examining people's use of preventative medicine, disease detection/diagnostic services and lifestyle behaviours. The core constructs of the HBM (Figure 4.1) are *perceived susceptibility* (to the disease or health problem), *perceived severity* (of the disease or health problem), *perceived benefits* and *perceived barriers* (in relation to the health behaviour), and *cues to action* (the prompt for behaviour change), with a later addition of *self-efficacy* (the control one has over one's behaviour). The HBM has been applied mostly to conditions where beliefs are more important than overt symptoms, such as in early cancer detection, blood pressure screening, other asymptomatic conditions and health concerns that are prevention-related.

It is worth dwelling on the concept of self-efficacy here, not least of all because it also forms a core part of the next theory discussed below. Imagine straight arrows joining 'person' to 'behaviour' to 'outcome' (Figure 4.2). While the concept of outcome expectancy relates to beliefs about whether a *behaviour* will lead to a particular *outcome*, the concept of self-efficacy (or efficacy expectation) relates to whether the *person* thinks they can perform the *behaviour* in the first place. Self-efficacy here is an individual's personal conviction about their ability to change their behaviour in light of their own

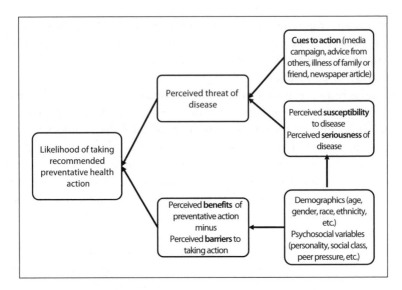

Figure 4.1   The core constructs of the health belief model. (Data from Becker and Maiman 1975.)

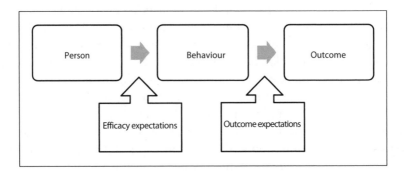

Figure 4.2   The concept of self-efficacy (efficacy expectations). (Data from Rosenstock *et al.* 1988.)

beliefs and circumstances. For example, believing that eating less will result in weight loss is one thing (behaviour-outcome) but self-belief about one's ability to eat less is quite another (person-behaviour).

Social cognitive theory

Social cognitive theory (SCT), initially labelled social learning theory, was developed by Albert Bandura. It too asserts that behaviour is determined by expectancies and incentives. A fundamental assertion of SCT is that people learn through their own experiences, as well as through observing the actions of others and the ensuing results (Bandura 2004). The core determinants of SCT include:

- knowledge (of health risks and benefits of health practices)
- perceived self-efficacy (the control that one can exert over one's health habits)
- outcome expectations (the expected costs and benefits relating to different health habits)
- health goals (plans and strategies people set themselves)
- perceived facilitators and impediments to change (Figure 4.3).

Knowledge features as part of SCT because ignorance, for example, about the impact of an unhealthy lifestyle habit on health, will produce little incentive for change. Beliefs about self-efficacy play a major role in SCT – unless the individual believes they can achieve a desired change through their actions, they will have little motivation to change their behaviour and so will persist in conducting that behaviour. The individual must therefore have the belief that it is in their power to change, in order to bring about a positive change in their behaviour. Of course, the outcomes of health behaviours are also important, so SCT also considers that the outcome people expect will act to guide their behaviour or intention to change their behaviour. Outcome expectations can include physical outcomes such as pleasure or pain and accompanying losses and wins. It can also include the social reaction evoked by the behaviour, for example, others' approval or disapproval. The final outcome expectation concerns one's own self-evaluation of the health behaviour or health status, for example, whether a change would boost self-esteem and self-satisfaction.

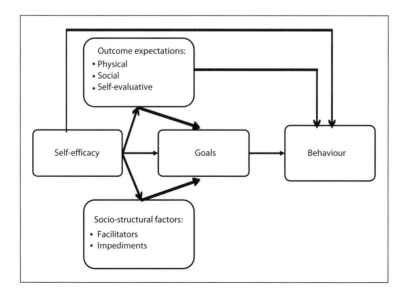

Figure 4.3 Social cognitive theory. (Data from Bandura 2004.)

People's personal goals, which relate to their value system, also influence people's health-related behaviour according to SCT. Here, it is generally thought that short-term goals that are achievable are most helpful in guiding people's action in the immediate term. The final features of SCT, perceived facilitators and obstacles, impact on health habits via their interaction with self-efficacy beliefs. Socioenvironmental factors can be judged to facilitate or obstruct healthy behaviour by the individual, so, for example, regular outdoor exercise might be deemed impossible because the British weather is seen as a real, insurmountable barrier to change. Economic barriers could also exist, including the structure and function of health services, which could be outside of the sphere of an individual's control.

Observational learning, reinforcement, self-control and self-efficacy are all thought to be important elements of any behaviour-change intervention based on SCT. For example, an intervention based on SCT would include goal-setting and self-monitoring as key components. Self-efficacy, which as explained above is an individual's belief and confidence in their ability to change their behaviour and take action, is a particularly important element of SCT. Thus certain strategies can be used to help boost self-efficacy beliefs including: setting small, realisable goals; using formal contracts to specify goals and rewards; and monitoring and support, including record keeping by the individual. In addition, according to SCT, role models and positive support can also be incorporated into a programme for behaviour change.

Integrative model of behavioural prediction

The *integrative model of behavioural change* (IM) is a theoretical approach to the prediction and understanding of human behaviour that is also applied in medical and health contexts. This model is in fact the latest formulation of the *reasoned action approach* (RAA), which includes the *theory of reasoned action* (TRA) and the *theory of planned behaviour* (TPB). According to its co-creator, Martin Fishbein (the other co-creator being Icek Ajzen), the reasoned action approach attempts to identify a limited set of variables that can account for health-related behaviour (Fishbein 2008). This set of variables can be applied to behaviour performed by healthcare professionals, for example, when deciding which intervention is best for the patient, as well as to the behaviour of patients and members of the public who are increasingly asked to participate in shared decision making and in preventative health behaviour, such as exercise or smoking cessation. Fishbein believes seven major variables are important in relation to health behaviour (Figure 4.4):

- *intention*
- *attitude*
- *perceived norms*
- *self-efficacy or perceived behavioural control*

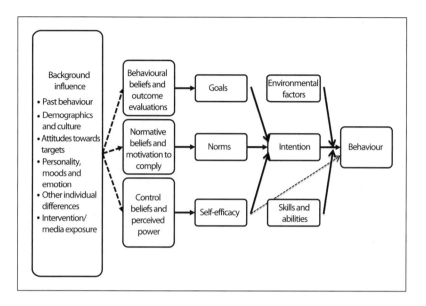

Figure 4.4   A reasoned action approach. (Data from Fishbein 2008.)

- *behavioural beliefs* (otherwise known as outcome expectancies or cost–benefits)
- *normative beliefs*
- *control beliefs.*

The RAA assumes that people's behaviour follows their beliefs about performing that behaviour. It takes for granted that human behaviour is rational and that behaviour can be described as reasoned. The first step in using the approach is to define the behaviour of interest, recognising that there is a difference between specific behaviours (e.g., eat a low-calorie meal for lunch during the week), behavioural categories (e.g., diet), and goals (e.g., lose weight). This is because, as examined below, it is generally easier to predict whether someone will engage in a particular behaviour than whether they will engage in a category of behaviours or indeed achieve their goal. RAA considers behaviour according to four elements of an *action* directed at a *target*, performed in a given *context*, at a certain point in *time*. For example, one might be interested in predicting whether a patient will always eat a low-calorie meal during lunch for the next four weeks. One way of defining this behaviour would be to state that the action is 'eating low calorie', the target is 'meal', the context is 'lunch' and the time is 'for the four-week period'.

The basis of RAA then is that the best predictor of whether or not someone will perform a certain behaviour is their intention to perform that behaviour – intention being readiness to engage in the behaviour. According to Fishbein (2008), many studies have substantiated the predictive validity of behavioural intentions, with meta-analyses reporting mean intention–behaviour correlations ranging from 0.47 to 0.62. However, intentions to reach *goals* (e.g., to lose 15 kg of weight) are only weak predictors of actual achievement of the goal because performing the behaviour might not necessarily produce the desired outcome.

In addition, the intention to engage in a *category of behaviour* is again not necessarily a good predictor of whether someone does engage in that category of behaviour. This has been attributed by Fishbein (2008) to differing definitions of behavioural categories such as dieting and exercising. Thus, according to RAA the most effective behavioural change interventions will be directed at changing *very specific behaviours* rather than categories of behaviour or goals. For example, helping patients change their intentions to 'eat more healthy food' or their intentions to reach a goal such as 'improving their physique' are unlikely to influence any specific behaviour. By contrast, increasing intentions to 'eat only a healthy, green salad for lunch every day' should increase the frequency with which the person eats only healthy salads for lunch.

As is clear from the intention–behaviour correlations quoted above, intentions do not always predict corresponding behaviours. This is because despite a positive intention, different factors might prevent an individual from acting upon their intentions. For example, the person might not have the necessary skills or abilities to perform the behaviour, or they may run into unexpected problems or environmental constraints. Clearly then, different interventions are needed to help people who have no intention to change their behaviour compared with people who have every intention but no means to act on the intention. Thus, if the idea is to change people's behaviour through a bespoke health programme, it will not suffice to develop interventions that focus purely on providing information and attempting to change attitudes, if the intended target already has the correct attitude but simply lacks the wherewithal (e.g., skills and abilities) to act on the good intentions or if there are barriers that prevent them from doing so. This would be akin to 'preaching to the converted' and any intervention in this situation would need instead to build skills or help overcome the barriers.

But if the aim is indeed to change behavioural intentions, according to RAA, there are three attitudinal determinants (of health intentions) that must be considered: the attitude towards performing the behaviour; the amount of social pressure felt in terms of performing the behaviour (normative influences); and the personal beliefs regarding skills and abilities to perform the behaviour (self-efficacy). The weighting of the importance of these elements in influencing intentions will be different with different behaviours and different patient populations. Thus while one type of behaviour may be totally driven by normative influences, another may be driven mainly by attitudinal considerations – and these may differ in different cultures.

The RAA requires the identification of the relative effect of attitudinal, normative or self-efficacy elements in influencing the desired behaviour in the population for which an intervention is being designed (Fishbein 2008). This is because, according to the theory, tackling the different elements requires different approaches, and for increased effectiveness the element that has the most influence should actually be tackled.

For example, the three predictors of behaviour, namely attitudes, perceived norms (social pressure) and perceived control (self-efficacy), when measured using questionnaires, may well be shown together to correlate with people's intentions to engage in six different health behaviours. However, Fishbein (2008) explains that closer examination has shown that the contribution of each predictor on its own is not the same for each of the six behaviours. For example, social pressure (perceived norms) on its own has very little influence on people's intention to exercise, while social pressure is strongly correlated with the intention to undergo a colonoscopy. Thus according to the RAA, although an intervention designed to increase social pressure in relation to the desired behaviour may help with encouraging colonoscopy attendance, it is unlikely to influence intentions to exercise.

The RAA is a normative model – it assumes an algebraic relationship between the different components, as though human decisions can be modelled akin to a mathematical calculation. The model assumes that the three elements of attitudes, normative beliefs and self-efficacy stem from underlying beliefs specific to the behaviour in question. For example, attitudes towards performing a particular behaviour are thought to stem from beliefs about that behaviour, perceptions about social pressure follow from beliefs about others' engagement in and views about that behaviour, and perceived self-control in terms of engaging the behaviour stem from personal beliefs about the ability to perform the behaviour. Thus, according to Fishbein (2008), it does not suffice merely to measure attitudes, perceived norms and self-efficacy – instead health professionals must identify the important underlying beliefs that lead to these outlooks. In another example, Fishbein (2008) explains that, although attitudes (rather than perceived norms and self-efficacy) predict adolescent intentions to engage in underage sexual intercourse, it is not merely attitudes that must be tackled but the specific underlying beliefs. So while 'intenders' have more positive beliefs about having sexual intercourse (e.g., will increase intimacy with partner or provide personal pleasure), 'non-intenders' have more negative beliefs about the behaviour (e.g., will result in sexually transmitted disease or make parents angry). Thus an intervention may attempt to either increase beliefs in the more negative outcomes or decrease beliefs in the more positive outcomes.

The RAA does not consider that the many other person-specific variables such as personality, mood, gender, culture and other demographics necessarily have a relationship with any given behaviour but considers instead that these act to inform the underlying belief structures indirectly affecting attitudes, norms and self-efficacy. That is, for example, gender or age may impact in one way on beliefs about performing a particular behaviour but in another way with a different behaviour. The challenge then is to design communications and other types of interventions that will successfully change or reinforce people's beliefs (which have been established and mapped using the RAA, for example) and to then explore the acceptance or rejection of these types of communication.

Transtheoretical model of behavioural change

According to its co-creator, James Prochaska (the other co-creator being Carlo DiClemente) the transtheoretical model (TTM) of behavioural change has 'stages of change' at its core (Prochaska 2008). The model considers behavioural change as a course of action that progresses through stages of change to include:

- *precontemplation*
- *contemplation*
- *preparation*
- *action*
- *maintenance*
- *termination*.

Rather than thinking about change as a sudden event (e.g., the patient will suddenly switch to a low-calorie diet), the model breaks down the process of adapting to change into distinct elements (Figure 4.5).

Precontemplation describes an initial stage during which an individual has no intention to take action to change their behaviour, at least not into the foreseeable future (e.g., next six months). A person may lack the information needed to make the change or may simply lack the motivation having, for example, become demoralised through previous failures to make the change. Such an individual will not normally engage in any activity that involves thinking about their behaviour as undesirable (e.g., smoking).

Contemplation describes a stage during which the individual intends to take action to change their behaviour (e.g., in the next six months). According to Prochaska (2008), the rule-of-thumb here is 'when in doubt, don't act'. Thus being in the contemplation stage does not guarantee the individual will take action but it does indicate they are at least thinking about it.

Preparation describes the next stage during which the individual actually intends to take action to change their behaviour in the immediate future (e.g., the next month). They may have formulated an action plan and have taken real strides in gaining some skills needed to make the change (e.g., buying a self-help book, talking to a health professional, consulting the internet). An

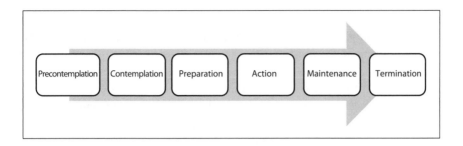

Figure 4.5 The transtheoretical model of change. (Data from Prochaska 2008.)

individual at this stage is considered to be a good candidate for recruitment to an intervention designed for behavioural change.

Action as a stage describes the actual modification of behaviour (e.g., within the preceding six months). According to TTM though, not all behavioural modifications count as true action – only those likely to impact on health outcomes.

Maintenance describes the period in which the individual is acting to prevent relapse to the previous behaviour. They may in fact be less tempted to relapse and more confident of sustaining the changes made to their behaviour. This stage can last from six months to five years.

Termination describes the stage where an individual is no longer tempted to revert to the previous risky health behaviour and unlikely therefore to relapse. In fact, the healthy behaviour would have become an automatic part of their life, like a good habit. This stage may never be reached with individuals remaining on constant 'maintenance'. Although these different stages are portrayed as linear, according to Prochaska (2008), the stages of change are dynamic variables that can be both stable and changeable, with the earlier stages of precontemplation and contemplation and the later stages of maintenance and termination being the most stable and the middle stages of preparation and action as the most changeable. Here an individual can progress or regress according to the help they receive.

The stages of change can be linked to thought and decision making by considering two main constructs: beliefs about the pros and cons of changing. That is, measuring people's ideas about the advantages and disadvantages of making the behavioural change shows a consistent relationship with the individual stages of change. This pattern of relationship has been found across more than 50 health behaviours as studied in 140 cases involving nine different languages. Thus Prochaska (2008) claims that while during the precontemplation stage, the cons of changing behaviour outweigh the pros, the opposite is true from the preparation stage onwards, with the difference between the pros and cons increasing at each stage. Interestingly, in the contemplation stage, the pros and cons are equivalent, reflecting people's indecision at this stage. Thus in theory smokers in the precontemplation stage, for example, can be helped to realise they are underestimating the pros of quitting and overestimating the costs so as to move them forward a stage.

Prochaska (2008) also explains that effective treatments can be tailored to suit each stage of change, the principle being to help patients set realistic goals. Thus, while someone in the precontemplation stage cannot be expected to suddenly give up smoking, they can be expected to move on to the next stage, that of contemplation. To do this, the pros of changing the undesirable health behaviour must be increased in the patient's mind. Once at the contemplation stage, emphasis should be placed on helping patients appreciate the pros of changing as well as decreasing their perception of the cons. If an individual in the contemplation stage is persuaded into a course of action without the change in the balance of pros and cons, according to TTM they may not be able to cope with what they associate to be the cons of the behaviour, turning contemplation into a negative balance which leads to discontinuation of the behaviour change. At the action stage, the perceived pros of changing the behaviour must certainly be greater than the cons. Once this positive decisional balance has been reached, however, Prochaska (2008) states individuals must be supported in other ways so as to help them maintain forward momentum. For example, individuals will manage better if they have supportive relationships with others, especially during periods of stress or difficulty that can normally trigger relapse to the unwanted behaviour. It also helps to adopt alternative healthier behaviours, e.g., during stress, to counter temptations to relapse.

Accordingly, TTM can be applied to change a range of risky health behaviours from smoking to avoidance of mammography, to medication compliance even. However, while TTM is an accepted concept within the healthcare field, commentators have noted the relative paucity of evidence for superiority of stage-based interventions over non-stage-based interventions. In addition, TTM assumes that people behave consistently and rationally. In reality, however, people can change their behaviour quite unexpectedly and without much deliberation or reason. In fact, the idea of the stages of change has been challenged by the notion that motivation to change is rather fluid and does not involve a sequential movement through the discrete stages. In addition, the model implies that active treatment should be withheld from those measured to be at the precontemplation stage – what if the model is incorrect and these individuals would have benefited nonetheless?

Fuzzy-trace theory

Both the RAA and TTM, as well as the HBM and SCT, assume analytical relationships between different elements of the models and decision making and ultimately engagement in certain behaviours, in line with normative theories that attempt to explain 'what ought to happen in a perfect model'. As discussed in Chapter 3, however, normative theories are dependent on a specific view of human rationality, where it is in fact possible to make an 'optimal' decision. It is also considered in Chapter 3 that in reality people can make decisions in the absence of clear information and these decisions can appear irrational to others, and so the explanation was offered that, unlike what is suggested by normative theories, people do not operate with machine-like logic, instead resorting to thought processes that appear to be reasonable to them at the time. In doing so, the idea of 'heuristics' was put forward; strategies that ignore some of the information to make decisions faster, more frugal, and possibly more accurate than complex methods. In addition, the interrelationship between emotions and thoughts was considered in some detail, putting forward the notion that that emotion too can impact on thought and thus decision making. If thought processes are so unpredictable, can an intervention ever be designed to influence change?

The fuzzy-trace theory (FTT) comes close to using many of the concepts discussed in Chapter 3, in a model relating to health decision making. According to its founder, Valerie Reyna, in considering judgement and decision making, it is important to first consider the representation of information by the individual (Reyna 2008). Two broad distinctions are made: *gist* representations of information as opposed to *verbatim* representations. A gist representation is a rather fuzzy and qualitative interpretation of the meaning of information. It is based on a wide array of subjective factors such as emotion, education, culture, experience and developmental level. Verbatim representation on the other hand is exact and quantitative, capturing the literal description (surface form) of the information. For example, if one is attempting to change someone's behaviour through a cardiovascular risk calculation, a risk assessment that returns a 10-year risk of cardiovascular disease as 25% will have the verbatim risk representation of '25%'. However, the gist representation will depend on what 25% means to the individual who is assessing its meaning. The risk could be interpreted as 'high' compared with an average risk of 10% (Figure 4.6). According to Reyna (2008), the meaning ascribed is dependent on contextual and individual factors that include even a person's ability to understand numbers. Thus FTT appears to embrace the concept of schema – that people draw on readily available mental representations of the world to interpret the information presented to them.

According to Reyna (2008), using gist-based intuition increases with an individual's development, intuition reduces risky health behaviours, and even that relying on *verbatim* memory can impair performance. In addition, according to FTT, although gist and verbatim representations are extracted at the same time, people prefer to use gist representations to make judgements

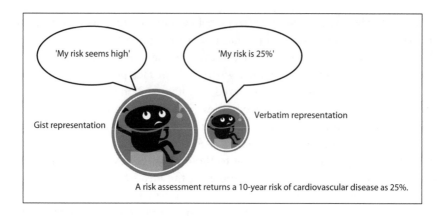

'My risk seems high'

'My risk is 25%'

Gist representation

Verbatim representation

A risk assessment returns a 10-year risk of cardiovascular disease as 25%.

Figure 4.6 Gist versus verbatim representations according to the fuzzy trace theory. (Data from Reyna 2008.)

and decisions – akin to the use of heuristics. This has important implications for health communication; although individuals might well receive and memorise risk messages in a verbatim fashion, it is their gist representation that will impact on subsequent health behaviours rather than the exact message that was delivered to them. According to FTT, people extract different levels of gist (e.g., categorical, ordinal or interval levels) from the information they are presented with and they tend to operate on the crudest gist level (categorical) as their experience or expertise increases. For example, the 25% cardiovascular risk might be interpreted as '25% is exactly 1 in 4' or with experience it might be interpreted at the crudest level of 'my risk is high' or 'my risk is high and I am going to have a heart attack like my father did'.

Whether gist or verbatim, the mental representation of information according to FTT does not in itself determine judgement and decision making. Rather, it is the application of people's values, principles and knowledge that determines the decision (Figure 4.7). So, for example, if an individual infers that they are going to *have a heart attack similar to their father*, they have retrieved knowledge about their father from memory, and applied it to the interpretation of 25%. By interpreting their risk as high, the individual may then decide to modify their lifestyle, for example, altering their diet and exercise level because they have retrieved the value 'better to avoid risk', in this instance, of a heart attack. Someone may have a competing value, for example, 'better to enjoy life while one can'. In this case, the relative importance of the values and whether they are flagged up in this context, will determine which comes to mind.

According to FTT, it is this integration of gist representation with the retrieved value that determines health decision making. Reyna (2008) provides examples of this concept with representations relating to undergoing health screening, using condoms, receiving chemotherapy, and even opting

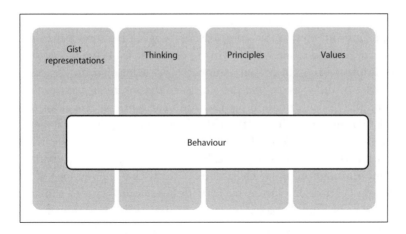

Figure 4.7 Concepts important to the fuzzy trace theory. (Data from Reyna 2008.)

for surgery to remove a lump. For example, if chemotherapy is represented by the individual as 'chemotherapy is poison' and this is accompanied by the cueing of the value 'poison is bad', according to FTT, the decision the individual takes will be not to choose chemotherapy. Similarly, if the intuitive gist representation of health screening is 'feel okay or take a chance on not feeling okay' (because health screening can return an unwanted positive test result), and this is accompanied by the cueing of the value 'better to feel okay', the individual will decide not to undergo the health screening.

It is in the context of gist representation that the processing errors, referred to as cognitive biases in Chapter 3, come into play within FTT. Because gist representations are key to FTT, it follows that the incorrect processing of information, leading to incorrect interpretations, can have a strong impact on decision making. For example, considering the framing effect, it is known that people have difficulty processing ratio concepts such as probabilities. Thus it becomes vital to help simplify processing by considering the manner in which information is being presented to people, so that instead of providing solely verbatim information, people are helped to make the correct interpretation of the *meaning* that is being presented to them. Gist information is important to FTT because Reyna (2008) claims that while people encode both gist and verbatim representations in parallel, they tend to rely on gist for decision making.

Impacting on the representation of information

According to FTT, one can help people make better sense of health information by controlling the presentation of what is communicated to them. This is especially so in the context of communicating probabilities, ratios and proportions because the verbatim presentations are not necessarily helpful on their own. To help, a graphical display can enable people to detect general relationships and make basic comparisons between the numbers being presented. For example, one way in which people can be helped to understand health information is to present numbers portraying risk differences using bar charts. In this way people can compare the height of bars presenting, for example, risk information for two different types of behaviour to form a gist-based understanding of the risk difference. Imagine that engaging in behaviour A carries a 25 (in 1000) risk of developing heart disease, while behaviour B carries a 10 (in 1000) risk. Rather than simply telling a patient this verbatim information, a bar chart could convey that the number of people developing heart disease drops by 15 with behaviour B (y-axis showing 10) relative to behaviour A (y-axis showing 25). The recipient of the information can then extract the salient point that behaviour B carries a 'lower risk' of heart disease compared with behaviour A. Stacked bar charts are also helpful as they allow the comparison of absolute differences rather than just relative differences. That is, including information on both the numerator (in this case, 10 or 25) and the denominator (in this case, 1000) avoids the overestimation of overall risk (Figure 4.8). However, FTT predicts that a visual display that only emphasises the numerator (showing only the number of people affected) tends to increase risk-avoidant behaviours compared with displays that also show the denominator.

Other helpful illustrative depictions of information include line graphs that show, for example, the development of trends over time (e.g., drug efficacy). With a line graph, whether the trend is going up or down, the message can be extracted automatically to help represent the gist of the information being conveyed. Another example is the pie chart, which is helpful for assessing proportions. And yet another example is the pictograph, where icons can be used to represent a particular population with a number of highlighted icons showing the amount of people affected by an event (e.g., to convey the risk of developing a side-effect) (Figure 4.9). It follows therefore that health professionals can use graphical means to devise decision tools that communicate important health information so as to influence health behaviours. In fact, Reyna (2008) argues that using relative risks, which encourage risk avoidance and preventative behaviours, should be favoured where possible to guide decision making that will result in positive health outcomes at population level.

Impacting on the retrieval of principles and values

Because according to FTT, it is the infusion of gist representations with people's values that guide decision making and, as per the discussions in Chapter 3, the availability heuristic operates when people make decisions, Reyna (2008) argues that retrieval cues can be used to impact on health

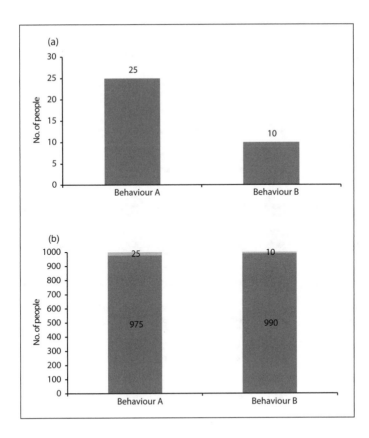

Figure 4.8 (a) Using a bar chart to convey the (hypothetical) relative risk of developing heart disease to make it evident that 'Behaviour B' is less risky; (b) using stacked bar charts to allow the comparison of absolute differences rather than just relative differences. (Data from Reyna 2008.)

behaviours. The retrieval cues are simple reminders about the risk of a disease, for example, sexually transmitted diseases (STDs) and the ways in which STDs can be contracted. The idea is to practise with a variety of likely retrieval cues until the relevant information is retrieved *automatically* in the correct context, rather than retrieval through deliberate thinking. According to Reyna (2008), it is possible to teach gist representations of knowledge, gist-based thinking, and gist-based values and principles through a bespoke health intervention, with an ultimate goal that participants understand the basis of a risk and are helped to retrieve and apply their own principles and values in the correct context to aid beneficial decision making. In this way, a behaviour-change intervention based on FTT would aim to help participants '(1) understand the gist of knowledge that will help them avoid or reduce unhealthy risk taking (which is expected to endure longer in memory after the intervention, compared with memory for verbatim details); (2) engage in gist-based thinking, rather than detailed verbatim analysis of pros and

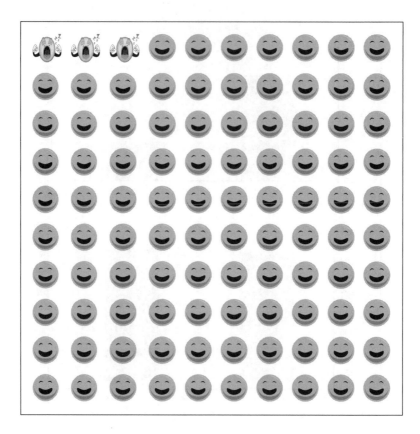

Figure 4.9 Using a pictograph to convey the concept that 3 in 100 people could experience somnolence as a side-effect with a hypothetical drug.

cons of risk taking; (3) quickly and automatically recognise signs that risk taking or danger is imminent; (4) quickly and automatically retrieve their core values and principles that are relevant in risky contexts; and (5) apply those values and principles to their representations of the situation to make healthy decisions'.

Impacting on the processing of information

Recall the array of judgemental errors and cognitive biases described in Chapter 3. Reyna (2008) has also derived FTT-based interventions that attempt to reduce processing interferences that lead to these mistakes in thinking when people assess health information. Examples of processing interference include the conjunction fallacy, the base-rate fallacy, the sample-size fallacy, and the framing effect. Reyna (2008) argues that these processing errors make it difficult for people to compare different information. An example can be provided via the framing effect where, because of the ratio/numerosity bias, people prefer a ratio to win of 9 out of 100 over 1 out of 10, because 9 is bigger than 1. There is also the frequency effect where people are more impressed by a ratio of 20 out of 100 than an equivalent of 20%, i.e., expressed as a percentage. With many of these cognitive mistakes, people are confused because they start comparing the numerator while neglecting the denominator in the information presented to them. Thus the remedy is to disentangle the information by representing it more clearly so as to enable mental manipulation of data when comparing them, using, for example, 100-square grids or 2×2 tables to represent probabilities. In this way, the recipient of the information can be helped to derive the correct interpretation of the information, rather than an incorrect gist representation.

Comparison of the RAA, TTM and FTT models

The RAA, the TTM and the FTT are distinct theories with clear differences, yet there are also similarities between these models (Spring 2008). To examine some of the differences first, the TTM assumes that the processes of change are generic and generalisable across a range of different behaviours, whereas the RAA presupposes that every behaviour is different from the next with specific predictors that are determinable. Although both the RAA and the TTM attempt to describe the normative ideal – what ought to happen with rational decision making – the FTT assumes that decisions are subject to cognitive heuristics, and that in fact intuitive processes are able to return decisions in context. In this way, RAA assumes that behaviour is reasonable and is based on thought-out intentions – that is, whatever a person's behaviour, it is logical in relation to their internal perceptions and objectives. Thus to influence change, one must target the strongest determinant of behavioural intentions (attitudes, norms or self-efficacy) for the particular health behaviour. The TTM on the other hand, considers the person's position on the 'stages of change' to be a strong determinant of subsequent behaviour. In this way, the TTM advocates different processes to aid change at different stages of change. The FTT claims that gist representations, the qualitative meaning derived from information akin to intuition, are the drivers of behaviour rather than literal verbatim representations – these are then combined with the values brought to mind to influence behaviour. Thus FTT advocates interventions based on presentation of risk compatible with gist intuition and drawing on relevant values so they can be brought to mind automatically in the correct behavioural context.

In addition, the RAA puts forward the idea that it is ultimately people's underlying beliefs that guide their specific outlooks – that is, the decision comes from a risk versus benefit evaluation. With the TTM, the emphasis is on people's assessment of the pros and cons of change at each stage of the process, with the product of this evaluation governing decision making. With the FTT the emphasis is on the dominant effect of gist interpretations, which override verbatim representations, and combine with recalled values to guide decision making – an ambiguous process compared with those suggested by the logical RAA and TTM.

To look at some similarities, it seems that all three of the theories accept that some aspect of the decision-making process might not be conscious (Spring 2008). According to the RAA, attitudes and norms (perceived risk) may not be consciously reflected upon to influence intentions and behaviours; according to the TTM, people in the precontemplative stage are unaware that they are 'underestimating the pros of changing and overestimating the cons', compared with the other stages (perceived pros and cons); and in the FTT the mental representation of information (perceived gist) operates automatically outside of conscious awareness. All three theories are also equally applicable to decision making and behaviour change by patients as well as healthcare professionals.

Application of theories to encourage changes in health behaviour

A number of systematic reviews have attempted to gather data on the use of theory in intervention design and where possible on the effect of these theories. Interventions for a whole range of risky and healthy behaviours have been investigated, which include fruit and vegetable intake and (re-ducing) the intake of dietary fat, screening for cancers, the prevention of injury, (reducing) sexual risk in relation to HIV and (promoting) the use of contraception. A publication in the 2010 *Annual Review of Public Health* examined the findings of these systematic reviews (Glanz and Bishop 2010). The authors noted that although several of the systematic reviews concluded that interventions based on theory were more effective than those not using theory, the mechanisms that explain the larger effects had not been studied. They hypothesised that the success of theory-based interventions may have been down to the use of theories that fit well the context of each study or sim-ply that theory-based interventions had been constructed with greater care, reliability and organisation. Most of the systematic reviews had examined small-group interventions rather than addressing organisational change or healthcare provider behaviour.

Whichever theory is applied in research, an important consideration is the manner in which theory is applied and the usefulness and external validity of the research for future practice. This has led to calls for more pragmatic trials and a focus on the generalisability and translation of interventions into real-world clinical practice. One systematic review of literature published between 2000 and 2005 identified articles that used health-behaviour theory along a continuum to include studies informed by theory (69%), studies that actively applied theory (18%), studies that tested the application of theory (3.6%), and finally, studies that built or created theory (9.4%) (Painter *et al.* 2008). Health behaviour theories are made up of a number of constructs and it is also sometimes the case that researchers fail to measure and analyse these constructs, therefore failing to demonstrate *how* the theory has helped change behaviour. Researchers have also been accused of picking and choosing different variables from different theories, making it difficult to ascertain the exact role of theory in the development and evaluation of the intervention.

Other commentators have categorised the current problem with theory-based interventions as:

- theory having been developed in an evidence-based paradigm rather than a practice-based paradigm
- theory focusing on the individual level rather than the contextual realities of the real world
- low accessibility of theories to practitioners who want to prevent disease through health promotion.

American academics and their partners have devised what is abbreviated as RE-AIM to 'evaluate and enhance the reach and dissemination of health promotion interventions'. Their aim is to encourage a whole variety of relevant people and organisations to pay more attention to particular elements of behaviour-change programmes to enhance the effectiveness and practical applicability of evidence-based interventions in the future. RE-AIM states that the five steps needed to translate research into action are: *reach* (the target population), *effectiveness* (or efficacy); *adoption* (by target settings or institutions), *implementation* (consistency of delivery of intervention), and *maintenance* (of intervention effects in individuals and settings over time).

Reach and efficacy are individual levels of impact whereas adoption and implementation are organisational levels of impact. Maintenance can be both at the individual and at the organisational level of impact. Further information can be found on the RE-AIM website (http://www.re-aim.org).

Conclusion

Most of the theories considered in this chapter assume analytical relationships between different variables of thought and decision making and ultimately engagement in certain health-related behaviours, in line with normative theories. The models each advocate different approaches to behaviour change. With social cognitive theory, behaviour change can be induced by setting small, realisable goals, using formal contracts to specify goals and rewards, and monitoring and support including record keeping, role models and positive support also help. The reasoned action approach, advocates smart, behaviour-specific interventions that increase beliefs in the more negative outcomes (of risky behaviour) or decrease beliefs in the more positive outcomes (again, of risky behaviour) while addressing attitudes, perceived norms and self-efficacy, as appropriate. The transtheoretical model considers beliefs about the pros and cons of changing behaviour at each stage of change to be important and advocates helping patients re-evaluate the pros and cons of change so as to move forward a stage. The fuzzy-trace theory is more in line with the idea of heuristics and cognitive biases. It advocates controlling the presentation of what one communicates to help people make the correct interpretation of the meaning of what is being presented to them and to reduce processing interferences that lead to mistakes in thinking. It also asks that patients are helped retrieve relevant information automatically in the correct context. In general, it is believed that behaviour-change interventions based on theory are more effective than those not using theory. Any theory used in a behaviour-change intervention though should be practice-based, ecological in nature, and easily accessible to practitioners who will want to apply the programme in their own line of work. While this chapter has examined health beliefs and behaviour-change models in relation to health (or health-damaging) behaviours, Chapter 5 concentrates on people's conceptualisation of illness and related behaviours by examining theories of illness cognition and issues relating to medication use.

Sample examination questions

Students may wish to use the following sample questions to aid their learning and revision before examinations:

1 Describe the health belief model.

2 Demonstrate the usefulness of cognitive models for changing people's behaviour.

3 Criticise the application of cognitive models for changing patient behaviour via a pharmacy setting.

4 Criticise the reasoned action approach as a model that could be used in the pharmacy.

5 Analyse the social cognitive theory.

6 To what extent is the transtheoretical model of behaviour change helpful to pharmacy?

7 Compare and contrast social cognitive theory with the fuzzy-trace theory.

References and further reading

Bandura A (2004). Health promotion by social cognitive means. *Health Education and Behavior*, **31**: 143–164.

Becker MH, Maiman LA (1975). Sociobehavioral determinants of compliance with health and medical care recommendations. *Medical Care*, **13**: 10–24.

Fishbein M (2008). A reasoned action approach to health promotion. *Medical Decision Making*, **28**: 834–844.

Glanz K, Bishop DB (2010). The role of behavioral science theory in development and implementation of public health interventions. *Annual Review of Public Health*, **31**: 399–418.

Painter JE *et al.* (2008). The use of theory in health behavior research from 2000 to 2005: a systematic review. *Annals of Behavioural Medicine*, **35**: 358–362.

Prochaska JO (2008). Decision making in the transtheoretical model of behavior change. *Medical Decision Making*, **28**: 845–849.

Reyna VF (2008). A theory of medical decision making and health: fuzzy trace theory. *Medical Decision Making*, **28**: 850–865.

Rosenstock IM *et al.* (1988). Social learning theory and the health belief model. *Health Education Quarterly*, **15**: 175–183.

Spring B (2008). Health decision making: lynchpin of evidence-based practice. *Medical Decision Making*, **28**: 866–874.

5

Psychological models of illness behaviour and behaviour change

Synopsis

In Chapter 4, health beliefs and behaviour-change models were examined in relation to health-enhancing (or health-damaging) behaviours. In the current chapter, models that relate specifically to people's experiences of ill health and disease management are explored. This chapter describes the influence of social factors but concentrates on people's conceptualisation of illness and related behaviours by examining theories of illness cognition and perception and their impact on illness behaviour and medication use.

Learning outcomes

You should be able to demonstrate knowledge and understanding of the following after working through this chapter:

- the role of cognition in influencing adjustment to chronic conditions
- the role of cognition in influencing the management of chronic conditions
- the role of cognition in influencing medication-taking behaviour.

Introduction

There are different approaches to examining people's behaviour when they are faced with an illness, and different stages in the process of illness can be examined. For example, there are the health-consulting behaviours; what people think and do when adjusting to chronic disease; and the behaviours associated with managing chronic diseases, which can include the taking of medication (or not taking medication). While a sociological approach may focus on the influence of social ties, social support and social conditions on illness behaviour, in line with the book's general approach, the current chapter focuses predominantly on cognitive models that attempt to explain the way in which illness is conceptualised and dealt with at an individual level. Although it is interesting and indeed generally worth while to learn about social influences on, say, patient behaviour, the focus of this book is on responses and behaviours at the level of the individual, where the pharmacist might be reasonably expected to have a level of influence through interaction with the patient in the pharmacy. Pharmacists can be expected to become involved in helping patients cope with chronic illnesses and associated management, and they might be better equipped to do so with a clear understanding of what affects patients' reactions to disease.

It is also important to make clear that, because of the burden it places on individual sufferers and the health system, the focus of this chapter's discussions is on chronic illness. Chronic conditions are more common with advancing age, and so it is expected that the financial burden they place will increase as the population ages. In terms of cognitive models, this chapter first examines Lazarus's appraisal model as a framework for understanding the role of perception and thought in response to illness and people's management of their chronic disease. People can respond differently to illness, adjusting well or, at the extreme end, suffering from emotional and interpersonal decline. In theory at least, knowing about factors that influence illness cognition and illness behaviour can assist pharmacy practitioners to help their patients cope better with their illness, for example, by addressing misconceptions and providing other support.

Clearly, for the pharmacy professional, it is people's medicine-taking behaviour (adherence) that is a particular topic of interest. Adherence, loosely defined here, is the extent to which patient behaviour matches the recommendations of a healthcare provider. A distinction is often made between intentional and unintentional non-adherence. With intentional non-adherence, the patient has decided not to follow the recommendations, whereas with unintentional non-adherence the patient either forgets or, for example, has problems with the packaging. Sometimes both elements may be at play. Non-adherence to medicines is a problem worldwide. The World Health Organization (2003) (WHO) last published a comprehensive report on medicines adherence in 2003. The report, not obsolete, outlined five key dimensions affecting adherence (Fig. 5.1):

- social and economic factors (e.g., poverty, illiteracy, access to healthcare and medicines, effective social support networks, cultural beliefs about illness and treatment)

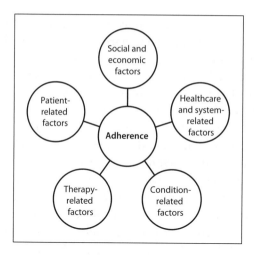

Figure 5.1 Factors affecting patients' adherence to medication regimen. (Data from World Health Organization 2003.)

- healthcare team and system-related factors (e.g., lack of knowledge, lack of tools, poor communication)
- condition-related factors (e.g., depression has a considerable effect on adherence)
- therapy-related factors (e.g., the dose frequency and the incidence of side-effects)
- patient-related factors (e.g., lack of information and skills, difficulty with motivation and self-efficacy, and lack of support for behavioural changes).

Admittedly, no one particular factor can be pinpointed as a leading cause of non-adherence and instead a multitude of factors are thought to work together to affect patient behaviour in relation to non-adherence. Nowadays community pharmacists in the UK are paid to engage in formal services that attempt to influence patients' adherence to their medication regimen via private one-to-one consultations in the form of the Medicines Use Review (MUR) and the New Medicines Service (NMS), the latter launched in the UK in October 2011. Models relating to medicines adherence and evidence relating to interventions that attempt to improve adherence are also examined.

Adjusting to chronic illness

A substantial part of Chapter 1 focused on evidencing the morbidity and mortality associated with chronic diseases such as cardiovascular diseases, cancers and respiratory diseases. Chronic diseases are 'illnesses that are prolonged, do not resolve spontaneously, and are rarely cured completely'. Chapter 1 also discussed that most of these conditions are strongly associated with preventable risk factors and individual behaviours, such as smoking, lack of exercise, unhealthy eating and harmful use of alcohol, and that these are behaviours that can differ according to people's social circumstances and social identities. Indeed as a result, the focus of Chapter 4 was to examine cognitive models of health behaviour and behaviour change so as to equip pharmacists with knowledge that could be useful in attempting to change people's risky behaviours to healthy ones, in an attempt to evade disease. But just as human behaviours are causally related to vulnerability to disease, so too are they related to the outcome of chronic conditions – that is, patient behaviour can also impact on their coping and management of disease. It would be wrong to think that the outcomes data presented in Chapter 1 are associated only with behaviours prior to disease. Morbidity and mortality figures also reflect different experiences and behaviours of people with a chronic condition. This is because, as stated above, people can respond differently to illness, adjusting well or adjusting poorly. How people adjust to illness and manage it can be a result of both social and cognitive factors.

Chronic illness can seriously disrupt the patient's life; it is not only the disease itself that they have to deal with but the impact it has on social functions, and emotional and physical roles. For example, people diagnosed with cancer, heart disease, lung disease and arthritis can have depressive symptoms to varying degrees at some point following the diagnosis. Patients diagnosed with chronic illness can suffer from fear or uncertainty about the future, experience pain, and have physical limitations as a result of their condition; clearly their life could also be threatened (e.g., by cancer). The impact of these factors on work and daily activities and the knock-on effect on people's finances can also be a source of worry.

Psychological adjustment to disease has been examined in different ways and a review by Stanton et al. (2007) provides a useful framework for understanding the breadth of processes and influences involved. Here, the findings of this review, which identifies three themes from the literature, are drawn upon: that chronic disease requires adjustment across different domains of life; that adjustment happens over time; and that there are marked differences in the way individuals adjust to chronic disease. Adjustment to a diagnosis of chronic disease involves multiple domains such as interpersonal, cognitive, emotional, behavioural and physical components, which all interrelate and influence each other. For example, depression and low mood can affect functioning and most notably increases risk of non-adherence to medication regimen.

Different investigators have considered adjustment to chronic illness using different theoretical frameworks. For example, Hamburg and Adams (cited in Stanton et al. 2007) focused on adaptive tasks that included maintaining personal worth, restoring relations with others, regulating distress and pursuing the recovery of bodily functions. Taylor (cited in Stanton et al. 2007) added the enhancement of self-esteem, preservation of a sense of mastery and achieving a sense of meaning to the cognitive adaptation theory. Moos and Schaefer (cited in Stanton *et al.* 2007) made other additions to this list such as managing pain and symptoms, negotiating the healthcare environment and establishing agreeable relationships with health professionals. These are all things that people do in their process of adjusting to disease. Others such as Spelten *et al.* (cited in Stanton *et al.* 2007) have focused on a functional approach, conceptualising adjustment as resuming paid work, routine activities and mobility. Yet another approach takes account of quality of life in the various domains of physical, functional, social, sexual and emotional life.

One important consideration is that culture, ethnicity, socioeconomic factors, gender, as well as personality, cognitive appraisal and coping processes can all impact on adjustment to disease. That is, people's thoughts, emotions and actions are important but they are situated in the wider context of their existence. For example, social change can affect people's social networks, in turn reducing social support and impacting on psychosocial evaluation of coping at the level of the individual. This chapter, as described above, focuses on explaining the cognitive models, namely, models that link individuals' thoughts and emotions to their behaviour towards illness. However, the social factors mentioned above are also examined, albeit more briefly, for completion. Another important consideration is that adjustment to disease is a dynamic process influenced by the progression of disease, its severity and prognosis. Although one may think of adjustment to chronic disease as something that takes place around the point of diagnosis and receipt of active treatment, for conditions that persist, adjustment can also refer to periods of remission, recurrence and end-of-life.

Social factors

In Chapter 1, it was established that social factors are strongly associated with health outcomes data and a number of diseases such as cancers and cardiovascular diseases, which are in turn associated with a number of modifiable health behaviours such as smoking, alcohol abuse and eating and exercise habits. But just as social factors and inequalities can impact on people's behaviour 'prior' to a disease, so too can they influence the experience of ill health. Those in less privileged social positions, perhaps because of lower educational levels or access to financial resources, can have greater depressive symptoms, a sense of helplessness and poorer functional status in chronic illness. In addition, culture and ethnicity can affect disease-related adjustment, with psychological symptoms having the potential to present differently across different cultures and ethnicities. Gender too can impact on the experience of illness, with women thought to report more depressive symptoms in chronic disease or greater pain, symptoms and disability in specific conditions such as rheumatoid arthritis. This could be related to gender roles, so, for example, over-involvement with others to the detriment of personal well-being has been linked with greater suffering from disease. On the other hand, companionship is thought to enhance women's quality of life and emotional status (Stanton *et al.* 2007). In the main though, because women often have caregiver roles, whether they are the patient or not, domestic responsibilities and household roles are thought to greatly influence the distress women suffer with a number of chronic diseases.

Another important social factor affecting the experience of illness is that of social resource and interpersonal support. For example, being married or having a large group of close relatives can both influence how people adjust. This is because adjusting to disease can require help from others, not only on a physical level but also in an emotional sense. Having others to provide support during illness can translate into a better coping strategy, in turn reducing stress in response to appraisal of the illness, for example, by allowing the patient to discuss and evaluate their illness in a sympathetic environment. Social ties can also be a helpful source of knowledge and can encourage positive health behaviours.

Of course, the nature of the disease and the burden it might place on those providing social support could erode the nature of these relationships and this is also an important factor in determining ongoing help and adjustment over a long period of time. For example, depressive symptoms in the patient can lead to irritation and dislike in those around them, in turn increasing anger between the parties involved and leading to reduced support. It follows then that unhelpful or antagonistic attitudes from others (which can include health professionals), social isolation or absence of support can also affect people's ability to adjust to illness. According to Stanton *et al.* (2007), in the Nurses' Health Study (a large cohort study), social isolation prior to a diagnosis of breast cancer correlated better with (reduced) quality of life four years following the diagnosis than did treatment and tumour-related factors. Additionally, in a study of patients with breast cancer and their partners, where patients judged their partner to be unsupportive or to be avoiding or criticising them, there was a correlation with patients' distress over time.

Outlook on life

One final point to consider, before focusing on cognitive models, relates to people's outlook on life. It seems that people's disposition, specifically inherent optimism, is also related to adjustment to disease. For example, those with ischaemic heart disease who have been assessed more optimistic after discharge from hospital have had fewer depressive symptoms a year on (Stanton *et al.* 2007). In addition, optimism seems also to predict recovery while in hospital and return to normal life following coronary artery bypass graft, while lower levels of pessimism can mean lower levels of pain 6–12 months following the same procedure. In cancer too, optimism benefits people with different cancers at various periods in the disease trajectory. How does optimism exert its effect? This is thought to be via better coping strategies, and use of social support as well as minimising negative appraisals of the disease and avoidant coping (see below for a fuller description).

Cognitive appraisal processes

Richard Lazarus's work was first mentioned in Chapter 3, when the effect of cognition on emotion was discussed, stating that Lazarus was a proponent of appraisal theory. That is, Lazarus believed that people make a cognitive appraisal of stimuli before experiencing emotion (Lazarus and Folkman 1987). In fact, Lazarus's stress and coping theory, which goes beyond looking simply at the relationship between thought and emotion, forms the basis of most disease-related models of cognition. To explain, Lazarus's widely accepted *transactional model* (interactional model) begins when the individual evaluates a particular event, situation or demand ('stressor' – e.g., a new diagnosis of disease) (Fig. 5.2). That is, one evaluates the situation's potential for harm and benefit. This primary appraisal of the stressor could focus on likely negative outcomes of harm, threat or challenge. An appraisal of harm means that damage has already occurred, an appraisal of threat refers to harm that might happen in the future, and an appraisal of challenge means the individual might see a resultant positive outcome as also attainable.

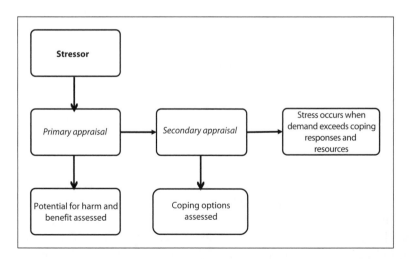

Figure 5.2 A simple, schematic conceptualisation of Lazarus's transactional model of stress. (Data from Lazarus and Folkman 1987.)

The model then moves on to explain a secondary appraisal where the individual defines available coping options for dealing with the perceived harm, threat or challenge. Here, one assesses the situation's controllability and one's available coping resources. The individual might identify coping options internal or external to them and these options may take the form of resources or responses. For example, a coping response for someone faced with the threat of reduced mobility (e.g., as a result of arthritis) might be to reduce their responsibilities whereas someone else in the same situation might take comfort from the availability of material resources to help cope with the same threat (e.g., enabling them to hire home help). According to this model, individuals experience stress where there is an imbalance between the demands placed on them and their coping responses and resources. But the model can change over time, as the disease as well as the resources and responses change; thus a different appraisal of the same stressor can result in less (or more) stress to the same individual in due course. In terms of chronic illness, perceived threats to one's life and goals, disease-related expectancies and finding meaning in the experience of illness are appraisal processes that have been most researched. These are explained, briefly, below.

Illness can interfere with one's plans and activities that normally bring meaning to life, and viewed in this way, illness can lead to an appraisal of harm, loss or threat. In fact, research has shown an association between negative appraisals of illness and greater anxiety, depression or pain in different conditions. In the same vein, patients who can accommodate their illness by altering their goals are less negatively affected by dysfunction brought about by the disease, compared with those who do not change their goals. Another factor that contributes to adjustment to disease relates to associated expectancies – these are factors relating to one's expectations (Stanton *et al.* 2007). For example, one's expectations in terms of ability to control the outcome of a disease can impact on adjustment to the disease. However, the problem with chronic illness is that outcomes cannot always be controlled or predicted.

Nonetheless, rather than giving in to helplessness, a sense of control has been shown to be associated with diminished distress, for example, in cancer patients. Whereas helplessness, say in arthritis, is associated with depression with some suggesting that this may, in turn, even affect the inflammatory process itself. Researchers have suggested that it is perhaps perceived control over symptoms rather than over the disease as a whole that is associated with the more positive appraisals and better adjustment. A closely related concept is that of self-efficacy in relation to disease, focusing on an individual's confidence in their ability to meet illness-related challenges. Yet another suggestion is that it is positive outcome expectancy (rather than perceived control over the disease, per se), or indeed response expectancy, that influences better adjustment in disease (Stanton *et al.* 2007). A final factor thought to be associated with the appraisal of illness relates to 'meaning' (finding meaning in life), which can be seen as a benefit of chronic illness, resulting in personal growth and enriching emotional life. Thus reporting personal benefit as a consequence of a chronic illness could as a minimum improve mood and the emotional impact of the disease.

Coping processes

As well as appraisal of an illness, the method of coping itself also affects adjustment to disease. An individual could direct his or her efforts towards approach coping or avoidance coping, along an approach–avoidance continuum. Those taking approach-oriented strategies are thought to seek social support and information, to problem solve and to actively attempt to find benefit in the experience, whereas those undertaking avoidance-oriented strategies might engage in denial and suppression and fail to engage appropriately in the process. In general, avoidance coping is thought to be associated with an inability to adjust to chronic illness. Of course, avoidance coping can also involve health-damaging behaviours such as continued smoking and this can hold back the type of behaviour needed for better adjustment to disease. Other approach-oriented strategies can include cognitive restructuring (discussed in Chapter 6).

Managing chronic illness

So far, a variety of factors which can be implicated in people's adjustment to chronic illness have been outlined, covering social factors, inherent optimism as well as, generally, cognitive appraisal processes. Next, Leventhal's self-regulation theory, which is otherwise known as the common-sense model, is examined in detail. This model provides a useful framework for understanding the role of cognition and perception in response to and in the management of chronic conditions – the model has stimulated a great deal of research since its inception.

Leventhal's common-sense model of self-regulation

Howard Leventhal and colleagues first outlined their common-sense model (CSM) of self-regulation in the 1980s. The model proposes that patients will decide to cope with illness and the threat of illness in ways that are consistent with their own understanding of the experience. According to Leventhal's model threats to health (e.g., perceived symptoms and illness) generate two separate sets of representations in the recipient: cognitive representations (an interpretation of the nature of the threat – illness perception) and emotional representations (an emotional impact such as fear or anxiety) (cited in Leventhal et al. 2008). These representations then lead the patient to attempt some form of regulation and management of the condition. So when a health threat of some form is sensed (e.g., via a primary appraisal), the individual will make a plan to avoid the threat or to control it. It is worth pointing out that as well as noticeable symptoms, a variety of other events can act as a stimulus for action and these include illness in others, and social and media messages. It is also worth pointing out that although the cognitive and emotional processing that form part of the appraisal process are listed as separate mechanisms, they do influence each other, as discussed in detail in Chapter 3. Another element of CSM is that the representations are thought to be appraised on an ongoing basis and can change in due course, meaning the model is about a dynamic process of self-regulation. Leventhal's model conceptualises people as problem solvers, who are actively involved in the management of their own health and illness. For health professionals, this means that patients can potentially be helped to achieve better health outcomes if they can be provided with a more useful understanding of their condition and the positive impact of taking on a more constructive coping mechanism.

Heuristics associated with illness and illness representations

Before moving on to discuss illness representations, it is perhaps worth while examining specific heuristics (mental rules) that people use to interpret symptoms of disease, and their underlying schemata. Leventhal *et al.* (2008) have identified four different classes, as follows (Fig. 5.3):

- the heuristics relating to an intuitive time-and-space mapping of the symptoms (for example, location, severity, duration)
- the heuristics involving patterns of symptoms relating to previous experience (for example, chest pain means a heart problem), novelty of the symptoms (for example, symptoms cannot be matched to existing schema), symptom trajectory (for example, symptoms are fluctuating or getting better), and control (for example, symptoms previously improved with self-care)
- the heuristics associated with cultural beliefs and social experience (for example, illnesses that come naturally with age or gender-linked conditions)
- the heuristics that involve active social comparisons (for example, whether the symptoms are as prevalent and severe in one's community and display the same characteristics).

Heuristics are important because people use them to elicit a meaning when they experience a symptom. For example, if a symptom has lasted a long time and is rather severe, it can mean that it is serious in its nature and could even threaten life. Such an interpretation could be reasonably expected to lead the individual to seek help in response. On the other hand, especially in the elderly, mild symptoms that have a relatively stable trajectory could

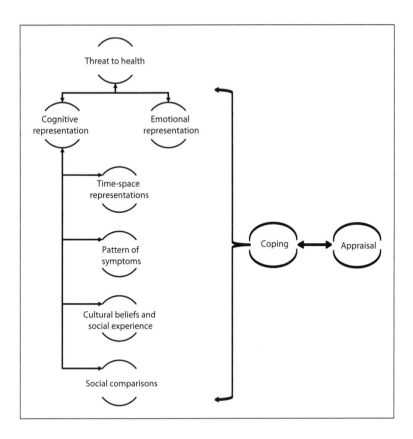

Figure 5.3 A schematic conceptualisation of Leventhal's common-sense model of self-regulation. (Data from Leventhal *et al.* 2008.)

be attributed merely to old age rather than a specific illness. For example, congestive heart failure, which is often accompanied by mild symptoms of fatigue, swollen legs and breathlessness, could be attributed to old age rather than related to the heart. Similarly, vague symptoms such as an aching body and general tiredness tend to be attributed to stresses of life; such an interpretation is unlikely to motivate the individual to seek medical advice.

However, multiple heuristics could operate so that vague symptoms that occur in conjunction with life events could be interpreted differently and could lead to care-seeking behaviour. Similarly, if heuristics join potentially unique experiences into one common interpretation, the individual might be more likely to seek help if they have an inkling of what the condition might be – a typical example is that of chest pain, sweating and pain radiating down the arm, which although unique as discrete events, together indicate a heart attack. Of course, illness-related heuristics are bound by the same limitations that apply to heuristics in general, explained in Chapter 3. For example, although availability and representativeness of health-related heuristics are likely to influence reasonable decisions, they could also lead to cognitive bias and errors in decision making.

There is also another point to consider. When presented with a set of symptoms, individuals are likely to ask themselves the question of whether they are likely to be ill or not. So while symptoms could match schemata relating to normal health, they can also cross the boundary into matching schemata that mean an 'illness'. That is, symptoms experienced can be matched to a label: an illness. This point is important in relation to illness representation: that to be sick is to be symptomatic. It means that patients who have certain conditions such as asthma will not consider themselves to have asthma when they are asymptomatic. This can have a huge implication in terms of adherence to medication for the prevention of asthma. In fact, studies have shown that people with asthma take both the reliever (e.g., inhaled salbutamol) and the preventer (e.g., inhaled corticosteroid) medication when they are symptomatic and not when they are not experiencing the symptoms of asthma (Halm *et al.*, cited in Leventhal *et al.* 2008). Investigators have even found the same pattern of behaviour in patients with HIV – lack of symptoms can mean patients stop taking their medication (Horne *et al.*, cited in Leventhal *et al.* 2008).

One of the most widely accepted models of symptom management relates to that of the acute illness model (Weinman *et al.*, cited in Leventhal *et al.* 2008) (Fig. 5.4). The model is a schema with five domains that are identified by the Illness Perception Questionnaire (IPQ), namely:

- identity (symptoms and label)
- time line (duration)
- cause (reason of illness)
- consequences (life-threatening or not)
- control (what can be achieved with self-care or medical treatment).

For example, with an illness that is represented by the patient as acute, management of the condition can be reasonably expected to alleviate the symptoms (relating to control) and the condition itself (relating to identity), will be time-limited (relating to time line); here the illness is non-threatening (related to consequences) and its management is linked to the underlying mechanism of the condition (related to cause). This explanation is why patients stop treatment when symptoms resolve or perhaps when other clinical parameters return to normal.

Treatment-related behaviours

It follows therefore that there are a set of implicit expectations associated with prescribed or even self-initiated courses of medication. These expectations relate to consequences, time lines, efficacy (ability to control the disease)

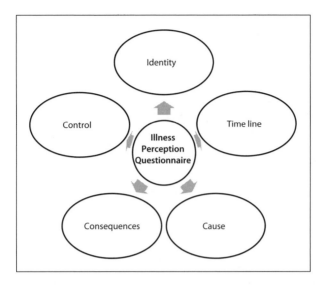

Figure 5.4 A schematic conceptualisation of the Illness Perception Questionnaire's five domains. (Data from Weinman *et al.* 1996.)

and route of action (causal explanation for effectiveness). This type of reasoning can mean that patients will adhere to medication that they perceive is controlling their symptoms, even if the symptoms are not associated with the primary condition for which the medication has been prescribed. On the other hand, researchers have found other evidence of conflict whereby patients with depression will feel that the medication is both working (causing side-effects) and not working (not improving symptoms of depression) against a background knowledge that antidepressants will take a few weeks to take effect (Leventhal *et al.* 2008). This type of thinking can lead to non-adherence.

How treatment is conceptualised is often associated with the representation of the illness itself. In addition, it appears that people hold a broad range of concerns relating specifically to medicines including, for example, that doctors overprescribe medication and that medication can be addictive (Horne and Weinman, cited in Leventhal *et al.* 2008). People also hold specific beliefs relating to the necessity of medicines and their harmfulness. Of course, these beliefs will differ with different conditions and researchers have examined patient beliefs about medication using the necessity–concerns framework devised by Horne *et al.* (1999) (Fig. 5.5). For example, patients with diabetes are much more likely to endorse the necessity of medication than patients with coronary or psychiatric conditions. Another example is that patients with asthma seem to have higher levels of concern about medication than other groups (Horne and Weinman, cited in Leventhal *et al.* 2008). The importance of these findings is that beliefs relating to medication

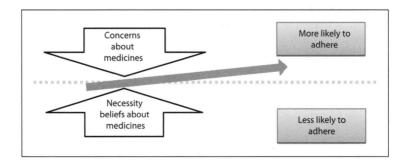

Figure 5.5 A simple schematic conceptualisation of the necessity–concerns framework. (Data from Horne *et al*. 1999.)

seem to be strongly associated with adherence to treatment, much more so than illness-related beliefs per se. This is such that patients with strong beliefs about the necessity of medication adhere better to their medication than patients who are highly concerned about their illness but do not see the necessity of the medication.

A related concept here is that of coherence and whether patients view the treatment as logical and in line with the disease. That is, whether there is coherence between the action taken to treat the disease and what the patient conceptualises as effective treatment. It follows then that patients can refuse to adhere to treatment that is inconsistent with their representation of the illness (Leventhal *et al*. 2008). Thus patients who believe that treatment is necessary adhere more to medication and, in addition, their belief that treatment can control their illness is congruent with a representation that their medication is effective for their condition. For example, patients with asthma who are adherent to their medication have been shown to represent asthma as a chronic condition and their treatment as necessary, whereas those non-adherent to medication have been shown to have concerns about treatment and believe asthma to be less controllable.

According to guidelines produced for the UK National Institute for Health and Clinical Excellence (NICE) in 2009, the evidence shows ultimately patients have a desire to minimise medicine intake where possible (Nunes *et al*. 2009). They may wish to do this to decrease side-effects and potential for addiction, to make the regimen more acceptable or for financial reasons. Patients may decide to use prescribed medication to improve symptoms or, deliberately, to replace or supplement medicines sometimes or all the time with non-pharmacological treatments. In addition, patients will make a judgement about prescribed medication for themselves by trying them and weighing up the pros and cons, considering the side-effects and acceptability of the regimen. They might even stop the medication just to see what happens, obtain information from non-medical sources and observe the effect of medication on others. What is more, patients do not generally disclose their beliefs and changes they make to their medication regimen to healthcare professionals. This is despite the fact that patients may not be able to recognise the difference between effects of medicines and effects of disease and, as outlined above, can have difficulty evaluating long-term preventative medicine where there are no symptoms. Finally, patients on multiple medicines may make choices between medicines.

Improving adherence to medication

It should be clear by now that patients behave in different ways towards their medication and that these behaviours are influenced by patient beliefs. It is estimated that 30–50% of medicines prescribed for long-term conditions are not taken as directed. A systematic review of communication about medicine taking and prescribing between patients and healthcare professionals published in 2004 provides some additional interesting insight into patients' concerns about long-term medication (Stevenson *et al.* 2004). As well as concerns about side-effects, patients were concerned that the medicines were not working, they did not like the medicines prescribed for them or preferred branded to generic medicines and even relayed rumours they had heard about their medication. It also seems patients have concerns about side-effects that they do not communicate to their doctor unless they are asked more questions by the doctor, for example. Where patients did express concerns, when they responded, doctors merely provided education or changed the medication dose or regimen. Now, if non-adherence is driven by patient beliefs, can providing education ever be enough to have an effect on patients' medicine-taking behaviour? If not, what type of intervention would help? This section focuses on adherence to medication and attempts to provide an overview of the types of interventions that may prove useful in tackling patients' non-adherence to medication.

A note about adherence-related terminology

It was mentioned in the introductory paragraphs of this chapter that adherence could be loosely defined as the extent to which patient behaviour matches the recommendations of a healthcare provider. This is because the definition provided in fact relates to the older term that captured this concept: compliance. The exact definition of adherence is 'the extent to which the patient's behaviour matches agreed recommendations from the prescriber' (Nunes *et al.* 2009). This is because in recent years there has been a move away from paternalistic doctor–patient relationships (which the term compliance implies) towards greater patient involvement in decisions about their own care (see also Chapter 6).

Another term to consider is of course non-adherence, where the patient's medicine-taking behaviour does not match the agreed recommendations from the prescriber. Non-adherence can be unintentional if it happens because of forgetfulness or another factor outside of the patient's control. Most of the discussion around patient beliefs and lack of adherence relate to intentional non-adherence, where the patient has made the conscious decision not to follow the agreed recommendations from the prescriber. It is important to clarify that as well as failing to take the medication altogether, the term non-adherence encompasses other departures from the recommendations including missing single doses, missing several days' worth of medicine or somehow altering the dose taken (increasing or decreasing it).

In line with the notion of patient involvement referred to above, another term has come about in the UK, which must be distinguished from adherence: concordance. Although concordance was initially applied to a consultation process that involved the prescriber and the patient coming to an agreed therapeutic decision, nowadays the term includes patient support in medicine taking as well as prescribing communication (Nunes *et al.* 2009). There's no guarantee that concordance will lead to improved adherence but the literature attempts to unpack what will improve adherence.

Interventions for improving adherence to medication

According to the World Health Organization (2003) report on adherence, poor adherence to medication is the primary reason for suboptimal clinical benefit of therapy. Low adherence is a problem in most chronic conditions such as HIV, cancers, heart disease and diabetes. One of the most comprehensive reviews of the evidence on the effectiveness of adherence interventions was published in 2008 as a Cochrane review (Haynes *et al.* 2008). The authors of the review stated that 'increasing the effectiveness of adherence interventions may have a far greater impact on the health of the population than any improvement in specific medical treatments'. Cochrane reviews are recognised internationally as providing the highest standard of evidence in healthcare via independent systematic reviews of the primary literature. This particular 2008 systematic review, conducted by Haynes *et al.* (2008), which was an update of an earlier review, looked specifically to summarise the results of randomised controlled trials of interventions that had attempted to help patients follow prescriptions for medical problems including mental disorders (but not addictions). The review looked at both effects of intervention on adherence and actual clinical outcomes. In summary, it found that for short-term treatments, 4 of 10 interventions in 9 trials had an effect on both adherence and at least one clinical outcome with one intervention significantly improving patient adherence but not clinical outcomes. This meant that less than half of the studies showed a benefit. The interventions in these short-term studies were simple on the whole, involving, for example, patient counselling.

The review identified considerably more primary studies that had looked at long-term treatment. For long-term treatment, 36 of 83 interventions (reported in 70 clinical trials) resulted in improvement in adherence but only 25 were associated with improvement in at least one clinical outcome. However, even the most effective interventions did not lead to large improvements in adherence and treatment outcomes. The effective interventions for long-term care were judged as complex, and included combinations of more convenient care, information, reminders, self-monitoring, reinforcement, counselling, family therapy, psychological therapy, crisis intervention, manual telephone follow-up and supportive care.

As well as the complexity of the interventions, the 2009 NICE guidelines on adherence provide a long list of reasons why it is often difficult to interpret interventions that attempt to improve adherence (Nunes *et al.* 2009). For example:

- studies are often accompanied by insufficient description of the specifics of the interventions
- there is a lack of standardisation in terms of measuring adherence
- interventions lack theoretical grounding
- trials are small in size and baseline adherence rates are not measured
- interventions are complex and labour-intensive and may not translate well into practice
- there is lack of clarity about patient involvement in the decision to prescribe
- it is unclear whether raters are blinded to the participant grouping.

Nonetheless, the authors of the NICE guidelines, having examined the evidence on adherence, were able to organise the data to answer a series of practical questions relating to interventions for improving adherence. Not all of the interventions were necessarily based on an attempt to address patient beliefs; nonetheless, the answers derived and presented are relevant and are summarised as:

- changing the dosage regimen
- lowering prescription charges
- changing medication packaging
- changing the medicine formulation
- using reminders
- minimising side-effects
- choosing mode of information delivery
- using therapy, e.g., cognitive behaviour therapy
- using contractual agreements
- using self-monitoring
- conducting medication reviews.

The first question related to the impact of changing the dosage regimen. Although there was evidence that complexity of a regime can increase adherence, the evidence was considered to be of low quality and the conclusion was that any changes to dosing regimen need to be conducted on a case-by-case basis. The second question related to the effect of prescription charges on adherence. Patients in the UK may have difficulty affording medicines and they use strategies such as delaying the dispensing of medication, not visiting the doctor or lowering the dose to extend the duration of the prescription. Although it may seem intuitive to recommend longer courses to be prescribed on one prescription where money is an issue for the patient, this in itself can cause problems because, for example, such a practice would reduce the opportunity for review of the medication. Thus no specific recommendation is made. The third question related to whether there was any effect of medication packaging on adherence. No conclusive evidence was found that medication packaging (e.g., blister pack versus tablet bottles) could increase adherence per se, and again the recommendation is that packaging should be considered on a case-by-case basis. On the subject of packaging, the authors of the NICE guidelines also sought to answer the question of whether the use of multi-compartment compliance aids (MCCAs) was effective in improving adherence. Although potentially valuable for patients with practical difficulties in managing complex regimes or for patients with forgetfulness, the evidence is not strong enough to recommend the widespread use of MCCAs to tackle adherence.

The fourth question posed by the authors of the NICE guidelines on adherence related to whether there was an effect of medicine formulation. Here, the evidence again was considered to be not strong enough so the recommendation is that changing the formulation of medication should be considered on a case-by-case basis only. Another area where no specific recommendation was made related to the use of reminders (the fifth question), for example, phone reminders or text messaging for improving adherence. This was because NICE did not consider that the benefit from any type of reminder was clear from the available evidence. The sixth question related to whether minimising side-effects via interventions improves adherence. The NICE guidelines, having considered the evidence, recommended a number of ways to manage side-effects to support patient adherence, including providing adequate information about side-effects, exploring how a patient wants to manage side-effects, reducing the dose of a medication and changing the medication to an alternative.

The mode of delivery of information to patients (e.g., written versus pictorial) was also considered (the seventh question). The NICE guidelines recommend that while no conclusive evidence exists, in some cases and conditions, the mode of delivery of information affects adherence. This should be individualised to each patient. The eighth question posed by NICE related to whether specific forms of therapy such as cognitive behaviour therapy (CBT), improve adherence. Again, the evidence was considered inconclusive for general application stating that patients make their own appraisal of medicines based on factors important to them, making their behaviour rational and coherent and thus not appropriate for CBT. The NICE guidelines also considered the effect of contractual arrangements between healthcare professionals and patients and found no evidence of impact. In addition, the value of patient self-monitoring in improving adherence was found to be conflicting and patient-group specific. Finally, the guidelines also examined the evidence for medication reviews. Although these can have benefits for the patient the evidence was found to be conflicting as to whether this led to actual improvement in adherence to prescribed medication.

How to improve adherence to medication

Interestingly, despite the apparent lack of objective and conclusive research evidence relating to interventions for improving adherence, the 2009 NICE guidelines on adherence provide very clear recommendations for improving adherence in practical settings (Nunes *et al.* 2009). Perhaps this is not surprising given the difficulty in translating even well-designed research to real clinical practice. In addition, the NICE guidelines and the findings of the Cochrane review need to be put into context. Viewed in a strict evidence-based context, the evidence for interventions that attempt to improve adherence is inconclusive. Viewed in another way, some interventions to promote adherence are efficacious but studies assessing these are perhaps not designed to gold-standard levels. Thus taking on board the body of evidence, a number of actions for improving adherence in practice are recommended:

- involving patients in decisions about their medication through better communication, information provision, patient involvement and elicitation of patient beliefs about medication
- supporting adherence through assessing adherence and making changes to improve adherence
- reviewing medication
- better communication between healthcare professionals.

Some of the detail of the recommendations is discussed in the next chapter, which focuses on better communication with the patient.

Conclusion

This chapter has focused on chronic illness and the way that patients think and behave when they have a chronic condition. It can be difficult to adjust to a chronic illness and patients often find their life has been disrupted in many ways and their relationships with their loved ones affected on multiple levels. People find different ways of coping with illness and how they cope can be influenced as much by their surroundings as by their inner thoughts and emotions. Inequalities can impact on the way people adjust to illness, and social networks provide an emotional buffer. Those with a positive outlook on life cope better with illness. On a cognitive level, Lazarus's stress and coping theory was examined. Illness can interfere with life plans but some people manage even to find meaning in their experience of illness so ultimately it is an individual's appraisal of their situation that influences their response. Leventhal's self-regulation theory provides a useful framework for further understanding people's cognitive processing in relation to disease. An interesting concept relates to the fact that people form their own heuristics about illness, which contribute to their perceptions about illness. When these concepts relate to medicines, they can have an overwhelming impact on whether patients take their medicines as prescribed or not. Thus the necessity–concerns framework, which attempts to capture people's medicines-related beliefs, was also discussed. It is ultimately the balance of these two components (necessity of the medication versus concerns about the medication) that is thought to direct patients' medicine-taking behaviour. Although formal studies have not identified any one type of patient that does not adhere to medication or indeed any one type of intervention that helps improve adherence, it is ultimately for the health professional to help improve patient adherence through better lines of communication and response. Whereas this chapter has examined people's conceptualisation of illness and related behaviours by examining theories of illness cognition and issues relating to medication use, Chapter 6 wraps up the theory chapters by focusing on effective ways of communicating and putting into practice what has been learnt so far in this book.

Sample examination questions

Students may wish to use the following sample questions to aid their learning and revision before examinations:

1 Define the concept of 'adherence to medication' and describe four interventions for improving adherence.

2 Describe the factors thought to influence patients' adherence to a medication regimen.

3 Choose an intervention that will help support an intentionally non-adherent patient.

4 Demonstrate the usefulness of Lazarus's transactional model of stress to pharmacy.

5 Verify the relevance of the necessity–concerns framework in relation to the work of a pharmacist.

6 Question the value of Leventhal's common-sense model of self-regulation in relation to the work of a hospital pharmacist.

7 To what extent is the pharmacist able to improve adherence rates?

References and further reading

Haynes RB *et al.* (2008). Interventions for enhancing medication adherence. *Cochrane Database of Systematic Reviews*. Art. No. CD000011.

Horne R *et al.* (1999). The beliefs about medicines questionnaire: the development and evaluation of a new method for assessing the cognitive representation of medication. *Psychology and Health*, **14**: 1–24.

Lazarus RS, Folkman S (1987). Transactional theory and research on emotions and coping. *European Journal of Personality*, **1**: 141–169.

Leventhal H *et al.* (2008). Health psychology: the search for pathways between behavior and health. *Annual Review of Psychology*, **59**: 477–505.

Nunes V *et al.* (2009). *Clinical Guidelines and Evidence Review for Medicines Adherence: Involving Patients in Decisions About Prescribed Medicines and Supporting Adherence.* London: National Collaborating Centre for Primary Care and Royal College of General Practitioners.

Stanton AL *et al.* (2007). Health psychology: psychological adjustment to chronic disease. *Annual Review of Psychology*, **58**: 565–592.

Stevenson FA *et al.* (2004). A systematic review of the research on communication between patients and health care professionals about medicines: the consequences for concordance. *Health Expectations*, **7**: 235–245.

Weinman J *et al.* (1996). The Illness Perception Questionnaire: a new method for assessing the cognitive representation of illness. *Psychology and Health*, **11**: 431–445.

World Health Organization (2003). *Adherence to Long-Term Therapies: Evidence for Action.* Geneva: WHO.

6

Communicating for effective outcomes

Synopsis

In Chapter 4, health beliefs and behaviour-change models in relation to health-enhancing (or health-damaging) behaviours were examined and in Chapter 5 people's conceptualisation of illness and related behaviours including medication use were examined. Chapter 5 ended with the consideration that although the evidence for the effectiveness of interventions for improving adherence is variable, nonetheless recommended actions for helping patients with adherence do exist, and are outlined in this chapter. However, no practice-based recommendation will be effective without appropriate implementation and communication at the practitioner–patient level. In the current chapter, some effective modes of communication are also focused upon. Chapter 6 explains a number of concepts including adherence-improving actions, patient-centred care and shared decision making, as well as the concepts of emotional intelligence, body language and cognitive restructuring.

Learning outcomes

You should be able to demonstrate knowledge and understanding of the following concepts after working through this chapter:

- recommendations for improving patients' adherence to medication
- the historical context of the patient–practitioner relationship
- achieving patient-centred care and shared decision making
- emotional intelligence, including emotional appraisal and the management of emotion through cognitive restructuring.

Introduction

Chapter 5 mentions that the National Institute for Health and Clinical Excellence (NICE) guidelines recommend a number of actions for improving adherence to medication, in practice. These recommendations are outlined. However, in relation to these recommendations and other behaviour-change interventions discussed in previous chapters, it is worth emphasising again that knowledge alone is incomplete without the tools that enable their effective implementation in practice. That necessitates a close examination of what makes for effective (or indeed ineffective) interaction and communication with the patient. The practitioner–patient interaction has always generated interest, and modern theories on such relationships can be traced back to the 1950s. Therefore studies of practitioner–patient interaction are summarised as a basis for ensuing discussions. Clearly, not every mode of communication can be considered in this book. The main emphasis of this chapter is to provide a toolkit that facilitates pharmacy professionals to communicate better with the patient, be it for managing feelings and avoiding conflict, or for promoting health behaviours and improving medicines adherence. The focus of the latter parts of the chapter therefore is on emotional intelligence and using communication cues for more effective outcomes.

NICE recommendations for improving adherence

The 2009 NICE guidelines on medicines adherence are introduced in Chapter 5. The recommendations for improving adherence are summarised as follows:

- Involve the patient in decisions about medicines.
- Assess adherence.
- Consider an intervention to improve adherence.
- Review medicines at regular intervals.
- Improve communication with other health professionals.

The guidelines recommend involving the patient in decisions about medicines through communicating better, facilitating patient involvement, recognising the patient's perspective and providing information. To do this via better communication, health practitioners should look to adapt their own consultation style, considering physical barriers to patient involvement (e.g., language barriers or disabilities) and adapting the mode of delivery so as to make the information more accessible to the patient (e.g., use of large font, or an interpreter), as well as encouraging questions and asking more open-ended questions to uncover patient concerns. Being aware that the consultation skills required for enhancing patient involvement can always be improved is also a useful point of reflection.

In terms of facilitating patient involvement specifically, practitioners should offer patients the opportunity to become involved in the first place, establishing the level of involvement they would like to pursue. The practitioner should explain the benefit likely to be gained from the treatment as well as the pros and cons of the medicine, at a level preferred by the patient. This should involve a discussion of what the patient hopes to achieve from the treatment and their own preferences, avoiding presuppositions about their views. Ultimately, the practitioner has a duty to help the patient make a decision about his/her treatment based on a clear understanding of the risk–benefit ratio, which should take account of different beliefs about the balance of these factors. Of course, patient involvement may mean the patient decides not to take the medicine or to stop taking it – this is their right so long as they have the capacity to make the decision (see box). If the patient decides not to take the medicine, the health professional should ensure that an audit trail is kept of the information provided to the patient on the pros and cons of treatment. It would also help to keep a summary of the discussions where the patient has expressed specific concerns.

Mental Capacity Act (2005)

To assess a patient's capacity to make decisions, the act's principles are used (http://www.legislation.gov.uk/ukpga/2005/9/contents). To lack capacity, patients must: (a) have an impairment of or disturbance or malfunction of brain and mind, and (b) demonstrate lack of capacity to: understand the information relevant to the decision; retain information for long enough to use it in the decision; use or weigh information as part of the process of making the decision; communicate the decision (whether by talking, using sign language or any other means).

The patient, their family or their carer should be encouraged and supported to keep an up-to-date list of their current medicines to include prescribed and non-prescribed medicines, herbal products and nutritional supplements, as well as a note of allergies and adverse reactions to medicines.

Similar to the argument in Chapter 5, it is now recognised that patients make decisions about medicines based on their own understanding of their condition, possible treatment as well as the benefits and concerns with the treatment proposed by the practitioner. Thus practitioners should first be aware that patients' concerns about medicines and their opinions about whether the medicines are needed will affect whether and how they take their prescribed medication. The practitioners should strive to ask patients what they know, believe and understand about their medication at the point of prescribing and reviewing medication. Patients should be asked specifically about any concerns they have about their medicines (e.g., to unravel any fear of addiction, side-effects) at the point of prescribing, dispensing and reviewing of medication, which the practitioner should address. Practitioners should also be aware that patients might want to minimise the amount of medicine they take and thus wish to discuss consequences of non-adherence, non-pharmacological alternatives, safe methods of dose reduction and treatment discontinuation, practicalities of taking each dose, as well as safe ways of choosing between a multitude of prescribed medicines.

In terms of information provision, patients should be provided with information in a format that suits their needs (e.g., logical and at the right level). Ideally, patients should be provided with information about medicines before these are prescribed, the information should be relevant to their condition and its treatment and should be easy to understand and jargon free. Relevant information should also be supplied at the point of dispensing. Rather than passively presenting the information, a discussion should be encouraged, taking account of what the patient believes and understands in relation to the treatment. The suitability of patient information leaflets (PILs) found in medication packaging is a hotly researched topic and it should not be assumed that PILs will meet the needs of every patient. The type of information that patients (including hospital inpatients) may require about medication include:

- what the medicine is
- how it is likely to affect their condition (its benefits)
- likely or significant adverse effects and what to do if they think they are experiencing them
- how to use the medication
- what to do in case of missed doses
- whether a further course is likely to be needed
- how to get further supplies if necessary.

Patients of course might not understand the information provided so it is also important to check that they have indeed understood what has been communicated. Patients can also be directed to web-based sources of information, for example, by referral to the NHS Choices website (www.nhs.uk).

After ensuring that patients are involved in decisions about their medicines at an early stage, NICE recommends medicine adherence is supported in two ways, via assessment of adherence and intervention to improve adherence. Finding out how the patient is actually taking their medication can help the practitioner make a judgement about whether the patient needs more information and support. Patients frequently take medication in ways that differ from the prescribed regimen and adherence should be assessed (in a non-judgemental way) at the point of prescribing, dispensing and reviewing of medication. For example, patients can be asked if they have missed any doses. Such questions should be:

- phrased in a manner that does not apportion blame
- accompanied by an explanation of why the subject is being broached
- focused on a specific time period (e.g., have you missed any doses in the past week?)
- about medicine-taking behaviours that include dose reduction, or stopping and starting medication.

A number of other methods can be used to identify potential non-adherence and need for additional support such as prescription records, pharmacy patient records and return of unused medicines.

Any intervention to support adherence should be considered on a case-by-case basis, specific to the patient needs, and could take the form of further information provision and discussion or practical changes to the medicine or the regimen. For example, paying for medication may be a particular problem, in which case the solution would be directed at options for reducing costs. Thus the practitioner should first attempt to establish whether any non-adherence is intentional or unintentional – for example, whether there are concerns or problems relating to beliefs about the medicine (leading to intentional non-adherence), or practical problems associated with taking the medication (unintentional non-adherence).

According to the evidence, no catch-all intervention exists that can improve adherence in all cases, so any intervention to increase medicine adherence should be tailored to the individual's difficulty with adherence. What would the patient prefer? Options for support should be considered together. Of course, the practitioner should attempt to address the beliefs and concerns that have resulted in non-adherence. In terms of interventions, the practitioner could:

- suggest that patients record their medicine taking
- encourage patients to monitor their condition
- simplify the dosing regimen
- use alternative packaging for the medicine
- use a multi-compartment compliance aid (MCCA).

If side-effects are a particular problem, practitioners should:

- discuss how the patient would like to deal with side-effects
- discuss the benefits, side-effects and long-term effects of treatment to facilitate an informed choice
- consider adjusting the dosage
- consider switching to another medicine with a different side-effect profile
- consider what other strategies might be used (e.g., timing of medicines).

The third major recommendation from NICE is to review medicines at regular intervals. This is because the initial decision to prescribe may no longer be viable, the patient's experience with the medicine may warrant a change or the patient may simply need support with adherence. When reviewing medication, practitioners should re-examine patients' knowledge, understanding and concerns about medicines, as well as their beliefs relating to the need for medication, offering to provide further information as needed. Patients should be asked about adherence when medicines are being reviewed and non-adherence should be accompanied by a clarification of causes and agreed actions. A follow-up review date should be agreed.

A final NICE recommendation for improving medicines adherence relates to better communication between health professionals, which is particularly important when care is apportioned or transferred between different disciplines and specialties and when different professionals conduct medicines reviews. For example, patients transferred between settings (such as hospital to care home) should have a written report of their diagnosis, a list of medication including new medicines recently started, medication stopped (and reasons), with clear guidance on which medicines should be continued and for how long, a list of known adverse reactions and allergies, and details of difficulties with adherence and action taken (e.g., provision of MCCA). The prescriber should be informed of any discussions about adherence and agreed outcomes when patients undergo a medication review with another health professional.

Practitioner–patient relationship

To appreciate the above recommendations fully, it is important to understand the historical context in which the recommendations are situated, that of less than satisfactory practitioner–patient relationships. This section draws on a review of the literature on the physician–patient interaction in the past 30 years (Heritage and Maynard 2006). According to this review, research dating back to the 1970s has identified the doctor–patient interaction as problematic, finding then, for example, that one fifth of parents of ill children left a consultation without a clear understanding of the diagnosis and nearly half without understanding the cause of the illness. Worryingly, a quarter of these parents had not reported their greatest concerns (e.g., because there was no opportunity or encouragement to do so). These communication failures were strongly associated with non-adherence to medical recommendations. Further research since has established a need to move from doctor-centred consultations (or practitioner-centred consultations to be more accommodating of other health professionals' involvement) to patient-centred consultations. Nowadays, all health professionals should aspire to operate patient-centred care.

Returning to the historical context briefly, one of the archetypal theories often quoted in relation to the doctor–patient relationship is that determined by Talcott Parsons who viewed medicine as a social institution with a primary aim to assist those that fall ill by returning them to their normal work-related functions (cited in Heritage and Maynard 2006). Thus (generally speaking) medical practitioners were seen as operators of a system of standard treatment techniques (universalism) who did not seek to make adjustments based on patients' social characteristics (particularism) and sought to treat patients without emotional involvement. According to this theory, patients in turn acted out a complementary 'sick role', which exempted them from responsibility for the illness and from their normal duties but necessitated motivation to get well soon rather than continue indefinitely in a state of illness. In doing so, the patient was obliged to seek help from a doctor and to follow the exact therapeutic pathway laid out for them.

Over the years there have been many critics of the Parsonian model, however. For example, Szasz and Hollender (cited in Heritage and Maynard 2006) noted that the patient passivity implied by the Parsonian model will depend on the character and severity of the condition, with some interventions requiring physically intrusive procedures such as surgery, while others necessitate self-medication and more active patient involvement (e.g., taking medication for hypertension). Thus patients cannot always be seen as passive recipients of medical expertise to the same degree. Quoting McKinlay and Freidson, Heritage and Maynard (2006) point out that Parsons' analysis of the practitioner–patient interaction happened at a time when medical authority had reached a peak, and doctors worked within a supreme profession that allowed them to authoritatively dispense medication and judgement. Freidson in 1988 is quoted as saying that Parsons' time 'was at a historically unprecedented peak of prestige, prosperity and political and cultural influence – perhaps as autonomous as it is possible for a profession to be' (cited in Heritage and Maynard 2006). Other critics of the Parsonian model have identified the 'medicalisation' of social problems as a particular consequence. In any case, the biggest criticism of the model is that it cannot be easily applied to chronic conditions that do not improve, no matter what the degree of patient cooperation.

In addition, according to Freidson, since Parsons' time the administration of medicine as a commodity and the shift towards medical consumerism have reduced medical authority and technical autonomy of the profession (cited in Heritage and Maynard 2006). This in turn has impacted on the doctor–patient relationship such that Parsons' model is no longer the ideal. It has always been recognised that the quality of the practitioner–patient interaction is of paramount importance. Heritage and Maynard (2006) quote Hippocrates in his Precepts (VI) as saying 'some patients, though conscious that their condition is perilous, recover their health simply through their contentment with the goodness of the physician'. It was a similar line of thinking that led to the call for a bio-psychosocial approach to medicine that will consider the interpersonal as well as the social aspects of the patient rather than merely the biomedical (see Chapter 1). According to Heritage and Maynard (2006), an influential critique of traditional biomedicine by Engel in 1977 (cited in Heritage and Maynard 2006) worked as the modern impetus for focusing on the practitioner–patient interaction. Nowadays, patient-centred care advocates listening to the patient fully, exhibiting care and compassion and engaging in other agreeable behaviours to improve patients' psychological, physiological and functional outcomes all at the same time.

Patient-centred care

Patient-centred care encourages focus on patients and their concerns rather than merely diseases and their assessment; practitioners are encouraged to see the illness through the patient's eyes. For example in the three-function model for the medical interview, Cohen-Cole and Bird advocate a data-gathering phase, whereby the patient's psychosocial context is considered; a rapport-development phase; and finally, an educational and motivational phase (cited in Heritage and Maynard 2006). In this latter phase, the practitioner also works to resolve any areas of conflict to negotiate an agreement on the therapeutic outcome. Thus, communication skills, empathy and involvement are prioritised over authority and paternalism. Of course, there are other models of consultation too, such as the Calgary–Cambridge approach (Kurtz and Silverman 1996; Figure 6.1), which advocates:

- initiating the session (establishing initial rapport and identifying the reasons for the consultation)
- gathering information (exploring the problem and understanding the patient's perspective)
- providing structure to the consultation
- building the relationship (using appropriate non-verbal cues, developing rapport and involving the patient)
- explanation and planning (providing the correct amount and type of information, aiding accurate recall and understanding, gaining a shared understanding by incorporating the patient's perspective, and shared decision making)
- closing the session (forward planning and appropriate closure).

Despite ideal models of interaction, there can be variations in practice. According to Emanuel and Emanuel (1992) the following dimensions can be used to characterise the share of power in the medical visit (Figure 6.2):

- who sets the goal of the visit (doctor, patient or both)

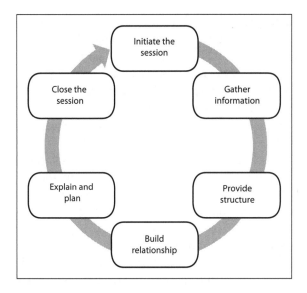

Figure 6.1   Salient points from the Calgary–Cambridge approach to conducting a patient consultation. (Data from Kurtz and Silverman 1996.)

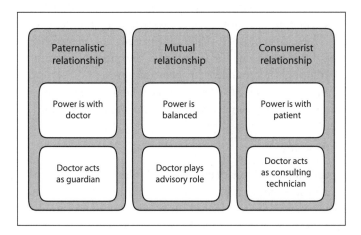

Figure 6.2   Sharing power in the medical consultation according to Emanuel and Emanuel (1992).

- whether the patient's values are explored (assumed by doctor, jointly explored or unexamined)
- the functional role of the doctor (guardian, adviser or consulting technician).

In a mutual relationship, power is balanced, the purpose of the visit is negotiated, the patient's values are explored and the doctor plays an advisory role to guide patient decisions. In a paternalistic relationship, the doctor holds on to the balance of power, controlling the agenda for the visit, goals and outcomes, acting as a guardian without explicitly exploring the patient's interests. In another type of relationship, the consumerist model, patients set the goals and agenda, making the decisions and determining outcomes with the doctor becoming a technical consultant. This line of thinking acknowledges that patient-centred care (the mutual model) may not always be achievable in practice. Indeed, some commentators suggest it is not always desired by patients.

Thus as well as advocating patient-centred consultations, researchers have developed various tools for assessing such consultations. According to Heritage and Maynard (2006), two general approaches to research include process analysis and microanalytic studies. Briefly, process analysis involves coding the practitioner–patient interaction according to a detailed coding scheme. A well-known method is that of the Roter Interaction Analysis System (RIAS), which is divided into socioemotional and task-focused categories (Roter and Larson 2002). Microanalytical studies 'deploy an essentially ethnographic and interpretive methodology to disclose the background orientations, individual experiences, sensibilities, understandings, and objectives that inhabit the medical visit'. Critics of the process approach point out that, although it can help to highlight the relationship between interaction variables and patient/practitioner characteristics, there is less focus on adherence outcomes, patient satisfaction and patient concerns. Thus coding in effect is thought to wipe out the sense from the medical encounter. On the other hand, although microanalytic processes represent the substance of the interaction, they are criticised for their subjective nature, which prevents the method from being incorporated in scientific, systematic studies.

Shared decision making

Focusing specifically now on decisions made during the medical consultations, and the process that leads to a mutually agreed outcome, the concept of shared decision making is considered. As alluded to above, nowadays shared decision making is advocated under the patient-centred model of care. Shared decision making involves a two-way exchange of information between the practitioner and the patient and includes a discussion of preferences for health states, therapeutic options and outcomes. Following this exchange of information, the practitioner and patient (and potentially others too) engage in a shared deliberation to arrive at a mutually agreed decision. According to the 2009 Health Foundation report *Implementing Shared Decision Making in the UK* (Coulter 2009), full patient involvement can be a complex process involving a number of steps:

- recognising and clarifying the problem
- identifying potential solutions

- discussing options and uncertainties
- providing information about potential benefits, harms and uncertainties of each option
- checking understanding and reactions
- agreeing a course of action
- implementing the chosen treatment
- arranging follow-up
- evaluating the outcome.

According to the Health Foundation report, shared decision making is appropriate when there is more than one reasonable course of action and no one option is self-evidently best for everyone: known as preference-sensitive decisions. Shared decision making then relies on two sets of expertise: the health professional is an expert on the effectiveness, potential benefit and harm of treatment options while the patient is the expert about him/herself, his or her social circumstances, attitude to illness and risk and values and preferences (Coulter 2009). Of course, both parties must be willing to participate in the process as the practitioner has to provide the clinical knowledge and the patient has to be willing to discuss their preferences. An extensive review of decision making in medicine and healthcare by Kaplan and Frosch (2005) concludes that although there is some inconsistency in the literature (some patients prefer a passive role), it seems patients are mostly interested in shared decision making but it is less clear whether doctors are willing to partake in the process. It seems that in reality doctors rarely offer elements of shared decision making in practice.

To help shared decision making, a variety of 'decision aids' have been developed. They can take the form of videos, web-based applications, computer programs, leaflets and structured counselling. Most decision aids share three features: providing facts about the condition, options, outcomes and probabilities; clarifying patients' evaluations of outcomes that matter most to them; and guiding patients through a process of deliberation so that a choice can be made matching their informed preference. Further discussion is beyond the scope of this book but Magic, the shared decision making programme supported by the Health Foundation (http://www.health.org.uk/areas-of-work/programmes/shared-decision-making/), the International Patient Decision Aid Standards (IPDAS) collaboration (http://ipdas.ohri.ca/index.html), and the Ottawa Health Decision Centre (http://decisionaid.ohri.ca/) all provide a good starting point for further information about decision aids.

So far in this chapter a number of concepts advocated for better communication with the patient have been outlined, including adherence-specific conversations, patient-centred care and shared decision making. In other sections of the book too, models purported to improve health behaviours are examined. The majority of this type of guidance focuses on processes that are thought to lead to improved care – in doing so, they cover the 'what?' question (e.g., what steps should practitioners take to ensure adherence?) and are predominantly process-based. The next section is devoted to an examination of the 'how' question – e.g., exactly how does one build rapport to engage the patient in a conversation about their medicines if they don't feel like they want to engage? As such, the current section draws on a number of specific theories and techniques from the field of psychology, all related specifically to the role of emotion in communication.

Emotional intelligence for better communication

As explained above, various communication processes thought to help with reaching effective patient outcomes have been examined. However, discussion of communication would not be complete without acknowledging the role that emotion plays in face-to-face interactions. Refer to the discussions of Chapter 3. Not only do people's decisions depend on their ideas about the world, emotional status can also influence decision making. In fact, there is interplay between thoughts and emotions – while emotions can affect thought processes, the inverse relationship is also valid. In Chapter 5 too, the importance of altered emotions, specifically as a feature of illness, was discussed. It makes sense, therefore, to dedicate the current section to a concept known as emotional intelligence. According to a comprehensive review of emotional intelligence by Mayer *et al.* (2008), the concept 'concerns the ability to carry out accurate reasoning about emotions and the ability to use emotions and emotional knowledge to enhance thought'. Accordingly, a number of abilities make up emotional intelligence:

- managing emotional responses
- understanding emotions and emotional meanings
- appraising emotions from situations
- using emotion for reasoning
- identifying emotions in faces, voices, postures, and other content.

Of course, emotional intelligence is closely linked to the separate concepts of emotion (coordinated responses to the environment) and intelligence (the ability to understand information). As stated above, emotional intelligence then is the ability to reason about emotions as well as the capacity to use emotions and emotional information to assist reasoning. Thus someone's emotional intelligence will invariably depend on how they understand emotional meanings. Such accuracy in emotional perception, or non-verbal perception, can include deciphering social information, such as power and intimacy relationships and accurate recognition of emotional expression, for example, in people's faces. Emotional intelligence can also involve being able to describe one's own and others' feelings. Emotion can help prioritise thinking and enable people to make better decisions or in contrast, emotion can bias attention so that more fundamental issues are ignored. Thus one particular skill is to be able to include emotions in or indeed to exclude them from thought, depending on the situation.

According to the four-branch model of emotional intelligence, overall emotional intelligence joins abilities from four areas (Mayer *et al.* 2008) (Figure 6.3):

- accurately perceiving emotion
- using emotions to facilitate thought
- understanding emotion
- managing emotion.

To explain further, an important consideration is the appraisal process that leads to an emotional outcome. The accurate categorisation and labelling of feelings is key in terms of matching a situation to a particular emotion. Although accurate appraisal may be a hallmark of emotional intelligence, misunderstanding an event or its consequences is not 'emotionally intelligent' and can lead someone to react inappropriately. Thus emotional appraisal and self-management become key components of emotional intelligence. These particular concepts relate to the clinical finding that one's emotions can become more positive by reframing perceptions of a particular situation. In fact, Mayer *et al.* (2008) conclude that emotional intelligence is correlated with greater life satisfaction and self-esteem and lower ratings of depression, and is possibly correlated inversely with some negative physical health behaviours such as smoking.

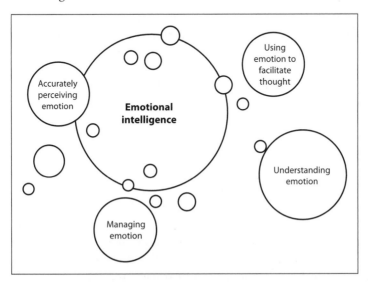

Figure 6.3   Emotional intelligence. (Data from Mayer *et al.* 2008.)

The next section will consider the two specific points mentioned above, that of emotional appraisal and also self-management by looking at concepts relating to the reading of emotion in others and the reframing of own perceptions through cognitive restructuring. Before it is outlined how individuals can try to reframe their perceptions, it is worth dwelling on what is meant by emotional misunderstandings. Recall that the concept of schema was explained in Chapter 3: people's generalised representations of social phenomena based on shared knowledge about perceptions of self and others, goals, expectations, events, roles, objects and memories. These well-organised cognitive structures influence the screening of information, its coding and categorisation, the interpretation of information and also the retrieval of stored data. Psychologists believe schemata and, for that matter, decision-making heuristics are a result of the brain's limited cognitive capacity. As well as being beneficial by making the brain more efficient, this type of information processing can lead to cognitive bias and the wrong decisional outcome. What can happen as another unwanted result is an emotional impact on the individual. Cognitive restructuring attempts to help people with the appraisal and interpretation of information, specifically to help with emotional management and can be helpful to pharmacists when communicating with others. First though, let's examine body language and the perception of emotion during communication.

Body language: reading non-verbal cues better

Body language and specifically non-verbal cues will be examined in this section, because these provide key information about an individual's emotional state. Non-verbal signals can include gestures, postures, facial expressions, gaze and eye contact, interpersonal distance, touch, smell and even the movement of the body – some of these signals will be focused on here. A range of emotions have been defined and there is certainly evidence that anger, disgust, happiness, sadness, fear and surprise have universal facial expressions – that is, they are expressed by humans in similar ways across all cultures. The evidence for the emotions of shame and interest is not as clear cut, certainly according to well-recognised researchers in this field (Ekman and Oster 1979). Although commentators believe universality confirms there is an evolutionary basis to facial expressions, it is important to consider that there are also cultural conventions associated with facial expressions, known as 'display rules' for managing expressions in different contexts. For example, people from some cultures smile more or show more control of their facial expressions or indeed are taught to substitute one expression for what they actually feel. Of importance to pharmacy and the health professions, students can be taught to clamp down on certain emotions and expressions and even to smile more and appear charming, irrespective of what they actually feel. It must be born in mind that the reading of non-verbal cues relies on viewing these as automatic, uncontrolled expressions of emotions but the discerning reader will realise that voluntary control and culturally defined display rules can also be at play.

Eye contact

As also mentioned above, non-verbal cues can involve more than facial expressions. In fact, to have any chance of accurately reading someone's emotions, it must be the combination of their behaviour that is considered rather than separate components such as the face or information gleaned from the eyes. Nonetheless, it is also worth considering eye contact briefly, as an entity. The direction in which people look is generally thought to indicate their focus of attention and interest and could give away their preferences. According to a review by George and Conty (2008), gaze (holding eye contact) plays an active role in interactions between individuals, presenting a significant signal for others to 'decode'. The gaze also provides an important indication of the emotional state of other people. Clearly, in a one-to-one interaction, say with a patient, mutual eye contact could be taken to indicate mutual attention. By contrast, averted eyes are decoded differently – for example, smiling faces with averted eyes are thought to be less happy than smiling faces with direct eye contact, while fearful faces are thought to be more scared with averted eyes.

As well as enabling an emotional judgement, according to Kleinke (1986), people's gaze can also lead to evaluations of liking and attraction, attentiveness, competence, social skills, mental health, credibility and even dominance. For example, continuous gaze is associated with ratings of potency, and there is the common belief that the ability to maintain credibility and truthfulness is affected by one's ability to hold eye contact. Certainly, in patient interviews, low levels of gaze (by the patient) can communicate non-involvement and in some cases even be an indication of depression and mental illness. For someone in the position of a health practitioner, according to Kleinke's review, there is a higher rating of competence when they engage in higher levels of gaze towards their addressee. The same applies to judgements about attentiveness, with higher rather than lower levels of gaze being judged as more attentive. It comes as no surprise then that gaze also influences people's liking of each other with studies showing that moderate levels of gaze are preferred over constant or no gaze!

Within the context of a conversation, eye contact can be used to regulate turn-taking with, for example, people starting and ending an utterance with a gaze. Here, gaze aversion (looking away) before an utterance is thought to help with one's gathering of thoughts whereas gaze after an utterance could indicate a desire for receiving feedback. Even the direction in which the head is turned during conversation can be encoded with turning one's head in the direction of the listener as a cue that it is their turn to talk and the listener's head turning away from the direction of the speaker as an indication of their own intention to speak. It is generally accepted that people gaze more while listening than while speaking. Again, in the context of a patient–professional interaction, it is interesting to note that people tend to increase their gaze when attempting to be persuasive (or for that matter, when attempting to ingratiate themselves). However, as already mentioned above, power, dominance and social control are also associated with the gaze, as is the communication of anger. In fact, by contrast, gaze aversion can be used to communicate compliance and conciliation. In this context, gaze can also be used to foster cooperation and bargaining as being able to sit face-to-face with someone influences cooperation better than telephone contact ever could. Those interested in more information about eye contact are referred to the Kleinke (1986) review.

Personal space

Another interesting and relevant concept relating to non-verbal communication is that of personal space, which fits into the broader concept of inter-individual distances. Personal space is the area that individuals maintain around themselves, intrusion into which can cause discomfort. Various techniques have been used to formulate standard distances that indicate comfortable inter-individual distances. Hayduk (1983) examined some of the methodological challenges posed by attempting to define these distances. Nonetheless, there are some generalised definitions of inter-individual zones measured as distances around an individual, intrusion into which causes some level of reaction, and as such, four zones can be said to exist (based on studies in the USA):

- The intimate zone (approximately 15–45 cm from the individual) is limited to intimate relationships.
- The personal zone (causal interactions) (approximately 76 cm–1.20 m) is reserved for friends and acquaintances.
- The social zone (approximately 2.13–3.65 m) is reserved for formal interactions and consultations.
- The public zone (from 9.14 m) is reserved for public events and public interaction situations.

These generalised definitions, however, fail to take account of differences in the size and shape of individuals' perceptions of personal space and their tolerance to intrusion of it. In addition, they fail to take account of context. For example, the size of the room and the activity the individuals are engaged in (e.g., queuing). What is certain is that there are cultural differences in spacing patterns. The founder of research into inter-individual distances

(Hall 1963), or *proxemics* as he called it, characterised certain cultures as having more tolerance to contact than others; for example, Latin-American, Arabic and Mediterranean people were described as having 'contact cultures', with Americans and northern Europeans as having 'non-contact cultures'. Similarly, Mexicans and Italians were said to prefer smaller spaces compared with Germans and Americans. People of Afro-Caribbean origin and Mexicans were also described as having closer contacts than Anglo-Americans.

Studies into cross-cultural differences in personal space are again beset by methodological problems and have been criticised for not being replicable. Perhaps the salient point to bear in mind is that people of different cultures to one's own will have different expectations relating to inter-individual zones and that the discerning pharmacy professional will look out for cues that indicate discomfort if, say, the social zone, is being deemed to be intruded within a one-to-one consultation with the patient.

Posture

The penultimate non-verbal cue for consideration here is that of posture, which can include body orientation, and is thought to indicate the attitude of the communicator towards their addressee. Body orientation is the degree to which a communicator's shoulders and legs are turned in the direction of their addressee (rather than away from him or her). Of course, body orientation can direct eye contact, which can therefore act as a confounder. However, some interesting results include that, for those sitting down, shoulder orientation correlates with increasing degrees of positive attitude towards the addressee, and that shoulder orientation generally can also be related to the status of the communicator to the addressee. Thus for individuals in the standing position, shoulder position is more direct with a high-status addressee than with a low-status one, regardless of attitude.

Another important aspect of posture is the openness of the arms and legs. Certainly studies show that people with closed-arm positions are judged cold, rejecting, shy or passive, whereas individuals who like one another are more likely to assume a more open arrangement with, for example, unfolded arms. Arm openness has also been related to status with studies suggesting an open arm position when standing is more likely with a high-status addressee, certainly with females. However, like most of the data making up the evidence pool for non-verbal cues, studies of posture are conducted in contrived settings and can produce conflicting results. Of interest to the pharmacy professional conducting a seated consultation, is that a warm attitude is felt by the addressee when the communicator leans forward on their chair, smiles, keeps their hands still and has more eye contact with the subject. By contrast, addressees infer a more negative feeling when the person communicating with them leans backwards and away from them on their chair.

Gesture

The final non-verbal cue for consideration here is that of gesture. Gesture has been defined as 'a movement of the body or of any part of it that is expressive of thought or feeling' (Kendon 1997). Gestures are thought to be more under voluntary control than not and the simplest examples include a nodding of the head to indicate 'yes' and a sideways shake to mean 'no'. In his interesting review of gesture, Kendon (1997) notes that, when communicating, individuals can use gesture in a whole range of ways to indicate anything from regulating each other's pattern of attention to the listener indicating understanding or assessment of what is being said. Gestures can also replace words momentarily forgotten to reach an understanding in conversation.

No speedy generalisations can be made about gestures except to recognise that in gesture, too, there are cultural differences with, for example, those from southern Italy thought to use gesture more than other Europeans. Interestingly, commentators note that the use of gesture has been viewed through the ages as denoting an uncultivated person, with restraint in gesture viewed as a virtue! It is outside of the scope of this book to detail gesture conventions but it should suffice to say that pharmacy professionals hoping to build better rapport with patients and others should also attempt to note others' (and in fact their own) use of gestures and the meaning being conveyed.

The field of non-verbal communication is vast and cannot be reasonably summarised in one section of a chapter. However, those interested in finding further information about non-verbal cues are directed to an excellent book on body language by Pease and Pease (2005), which covers additional topics such as hand-to-face gestures (which could indicate dishonesty!), palm gestures, handshakes, mirroring behaviours and much more. Written for the lay reader and not fully referenced, the book nonetheless draws on the author's extensive experience in this field and serves as a good basis for those interested in enhancing their ability to communicate with others.

For now, having considered emotional appraisal and accurately perceiving the emotional dynamics during communication, through the reading of non-verbal cues, the next section focuses on managing emotion and in particular self-management of emotional responses through cognitive restructuring.

Cognitive restructuring: managing the emotional appraisal

As discussed in a previous section, as well as appraising emotion from situations, and indeed using non-verbal cues to enhance emotional rapport, managing one's own emotional response is also key to becoming more emotionally intelligent. It is not always easy to decipher the right message or indeed to control one's emotions, especially when expected to remain emotionally detached as a health professional. Yet, cognitive restructuring can be an effective way of managing one's emotional response and can be used by pharmacists to help improve communication with patients. Cognitive restructuring is an approach-oriented strategy. It involves the application of certain techniques focusing on thoughts and actions, which have been shown to be beneficial in relation to coping. For example, people can be taught to recognise and learn to refute unproductive thoughts and actions. The foundation of this approach is that of cognitive theory, which links information processing with emotional, motivational and behavioural responses, something that will by now be familiar.

According to Beck, the founder of the current approach (cognitive technique/therapy), cognitive appraisal of a stimulus (whether it is external or internal) will influence the other systems (emotion, motivation, behaviour) and will itself be affected by them (Beck and Dozois 2011). Thus three basic guiding principles of cognitive techniques are outlined here. Some of these principles will be familiar by now but are stated here for completion.

First, individuals do not respond directly to their environment, they respond to their own cognitive interpretations of the environment. Second, and as discussed before, cognitions (thoughts), emotions (feelings) and behaviours (actions) are causally interrelated. Third, the prediction and understanding of negative cognitions and behaviours are enhanced by paying attention to personal expectancies, beliefs and attributions.

Put another way and to be fully effective, one can also consider the following propositions of cognitive techniques. First, that individuals, with training, motivation and attention can become aware of the content and process of their own thinking. Second, the way that people think influences their emotional and behavioural responses. Third, that people can change their cognitive and behavioural responses. This approach then, is based on an understanding that people, including pharmacists, can have erroneous thoughts, which they can be taught to put right so as to minimise the emotional impact of their thoughts.

In fact, a whole array of 'erroneous thoughts' have been identified and conceptualised and one of the main ways in which unwanted emotions can be better self-managed through cognitive techniques is to gain the ability in the first place to recognise that an incorrect thought has even occurred. Some examples of erroneous thought are outlined here but there are also easily accessible books that conceptualise these and cognitive techniques in more detail, such as a book by Willson and Branch (2006) written for a general audience. Erroneous thoughts can include 'catastrophising', which is taking a small negative event and imagining all manner of potential disasters resulting from that event.

For example, a patient might want to end a Medicines Use Review consultation quicker than you expected – catastrophising would involve you in thinking that this was an indication that your communication and indeed consultation skills are poor, have always been poor and will never improve. In reality, the patient might have just remembered that they are late for another important appointment. In another pharmacy context, you might be triggered to doubt the accuracy of a checking task last month (whose specific patient details you can't now remember) and go on to catastrophise by imagining all manner of negative repercussions, including being struck off the pharmaceutical register and losing your home as a result of being out of work.

Another example of an erroneous thought is known as 'fortune telling'. Here, predictions are made about the future, without any real justification. For example, you imagine that, because you did not score highly during your university OSCE (Objective Structured Clinical Examination), conducting your pre-registration year in the hospital will be a disaster because you will have a large range of people with whom to interact. This type of thinking stops people from acting as they should, creating a self-fulfilling prophecy! Yet another example of erroneous thinking is that of 'mind reading'. Although the section above was intended to help with deciphering emotional messages in communication, no one can fully read someone else's thoughts. Mind reading as an erroneous thought often involves thinking that others have negative motives and thoughts towards you. For example, a patient who always rushes in to collect their prescription might choose to park on the double-yellow lines outside but the pharmacist might interpret their hasty behaviour as a sign of personal dislike towards them.

One cognitive restructuring technique involves learning to assess the severity of a situation (e.g., new diagnosis of disease or negative interaction with a patient) in a different way by considering the perspective in which, for example, the diagnosis/interaction is being viewed. Here, individuals ask themselves specific questions when such a negative event is encountered. Say if a patient is devastated by a diagnosis of arthritis, they might ask themselves if the illness will be as severe as they first think, with the right treatment and in due course. Alternatively, following a negative interaction with a patient, the pharmacy professional might ask himself or herself if the encounter was really as bad as he or she imagined.

A related cognitive technique is based on the premise that people believe other people or events outside of themselves are responsible for how they feel and behave. The A-B-C model can be used to represent this concept, based on A being the activating event and C the consequences (feelings and behaviour) that occur in relation to the activating event (say an imperfect encounter with a doctor). Cognitive restructuring concerns changing the B component of the model, the beliefs that occur between the activating event (A) and the consequences (C). This is also in line with the interactional model of stress described in Chapter 3 and an argument that the appraisal of the stressor can be modified by the individual.

Taking the above example of an encounter with a seemingly unconcerned and cold doctor, using cognitive restructuring a patient would distinguish that it is not necessarily the doctor's behaviour that leads to their own feelings of frustration but their own thoughts and beliefs that mediate the response. The patient might see that the belief they hold (for example, I have paid for the NHS all my life, having worked hard so I expect that the doctor should be polite and empathetic in return) will lead to increased stress because the patient cannot possibly control the behaviour of other people, including a doctor. Restructuring the thought would lead the patient to substitute a more rational belief (for example, I am not responsible for the behaviour of this doctor; or this doctor's apparent lack of empathy is not related to my behaviour but to frustration with their own situation, perhaps long working hours). Ultimately, the goal is to tolerate stressors by replacing negative feelings with neutral ones or less negative ones.

Conclusion

This chapter has focused on communication. Recommendations for improving adherence to medication have been considered. Patients should be involved in decisions about their medicines, their adherence to medicines should be monitored and improved if possible and the patient's medicines should be reviewed at regular intervals. Health professionals should also strive for better communication with colleagues and others involved in patients' care. The practitioner–patient relationship has been studied for many decades. Nowadays, patient-centred care encourages professionals to focus on the patient's perspective on illness and a number of models exist to help professionals conduct better consultations. Ideally, a consultation should be a mutual relationship where there is equal distribution of power between the patient and the healthcare professional and where shared decision making takes place, if appropriate, involving a two-way exchange of information and a shared deliberation. As well as considering process-based recommendations about better communication with the patient, practitioners should also improve their awareness of the role of emotion within communication, to become more emotionally intelligent. Here, perceiving emotion and the self-management of emotions become key to better communication.

A range of non-verbal cues can be used to both read patients' emotional states and to project a desired emotional response within a consultative situation. Facial expressions, for example, can be manipulated to hide real emotional feelings, eye contact can be used for giving reassurance, creating confidence and guiding communication, inter-individual preferences for space can be recognised and respected to create better rapport, and finally, awareness of both posture and gesture can be used to read and express emotion better within the interaction. In addition, people, including health professionals, can be taught to recognise and refute their own unproductive thoughts and thus better manage their emotional response to certain situations. Thoughts, feelings and behaviours are interlinked and once individuals become aware of their thought processes, it is possible to learn to recognise erroneous thoughts and to learn ways of restructuring these thoughts to achieve more positive emotional responses.

This summary of the current chapter brings the theory chapters to a close. The next chapter is concerned with the application of the theories through case-based scenarios and tasks that move sequentially from undergraduate Level 1 through to Masters level.

Sample examination questions

Students may wish to use the following sample questions to aid their learning and revision before examinations:

1 Give a definition of emotional intelligence and use an example to clarify your answer.

2 Describe what is meant by patient-centred care.

3 Summarise salient points in relation to how body language could be used to improve communication.

4 Summarise cognitive restructuring as a concept, giving one example to illustrate your answer.

5 Analyse NICE's recommendations for improving adherence.

6 Choose the most important non-verbal signal in a pharmacy context.

7 To what extent is shared decision making important to the work of the pharmacist?

References and further reading

Beck AT, Dozois DJA (2011). Cognitive therapy: current status and future directions. *Annual Review of Medicine*, **62**: 397–409.

Coulter A (2009). *Implementing Shared Decision Making in the UK: A Report for the Health Foundation*. London: The Health Foundation.

Ekman P, Oster H (1979). Facial expressions of emotion. *Annual Review of Psychology*, **30**: 527–554.

Emanuel EJ, Emanuel LL (1992). Four models of the physician-patient relationship. *Journal of the American Medical Association*, **267**: 2221–2226.

George N, Conty L (2008). Facing the gaze of others. *Neurophysiologie Clinique*, **38**: 197–207.

Hall ET (1963). A system for the notation of proxemics behaviour. *American Anthropologist*, **65**: 1003–1026.

Hayduk LA (1983). Personal space: where we now stand. *Psychological Bulletin*, **94**: 293–335.

Heritage J, Maynard DW (2006). Problems and prospects in the study of physician-patient interaction: 30 years of research. *Annual Review of Sociology*, 32: 351–374.

Kaplan RM, Frosch DL (2005). Decision making in medicine and health care. *Annual Review of Clinical Psychology*, 1: 256–525.

Kendon A (1997). Gesture. *Annual Review of Anthropology*, 26: 109–128.

Kleinke CL (1986). Gaze and eye contact: a research review. *Psychological Bulletin*, 100: 78–100.

Kurtz SM, Silverman JD (1996). The Calgary–Cambridge referenced observation guides: an aid to defining the curriculum and organizing the teaching in communication training programmes. *Medical Education*, 30: 83–89.

Mayer JD *et al.* (2008). Human abilities: emotional intelligence. *Annual Review of Psychology*, 59: 507–536.

Nunes V *et al.* (2009). *Clinical Guidelines and Evidence Review for Medicines Adherence: Involving patients in decisions about prescribed medicines and supporting adherence.* London: National Collaborating Centre for Primary Care and Royal College of General Practitioners.

Pease A, Pease B (2005). *The Definitive Book of Body Language: How to Read Others' Attitudes by their Gestures.* London: Orion.

Roter D, Larson S (2002). The Roter interaction analysis system (RIAS): utility and flexibility for analysis of medical interactions. *Patient Education and Counseling*, 46: 243–251.

Willson R, Branch R (2006). *Cognitive Behavioural Therapy for Dummies.* Chichester: John Wiley & Sons.

7

Patient case studies

Teaching notes

Educational objectives

The purpose of writing these cases is to help you put the learning from the theory chapters into context via examples that mimic real-life scenarios. The idea is that you should be able to work through each case as suggested, to reach the desired learning outcomes. The main source of information for tackling the cases should be the earlier theory chapters. As well as being used for independent learning, the cases can be potentially integrated as part of university-led teaching, for example, in problem-based learning workshops. In addition, although the cases can be considered to be 'data rich', none represents particularly rare or unusual medical encounters. This is because the cases have not been written specifically to test your 'clinical' or 'legal/ethical' understanding – they are written instead to test your ability to apply the social and cognitive pharmacy knowledge presented in the preceding chapters. Although it is acknowledged that clinical or legal/ethical aspects might also be brought in for a more rounded approach, the main aim is to use the theory and case study chapters together as a self-sufficient learning tool. Finally, one important note is that although they have been written to mimic real life, none of the cases has been modelled on any specific patient, pharmacist or encounter and thus any resemblance of names to actual persons is purely coincidental.

The cases can be read by students at all levels of learning, although the tasks get progressively more complex – see below for recommendations as to which student grades might be reasonably expected to tackle each task. Generally, students at Level 1 (Stage/Year 1 of the MPharm degree) should tackle the first task while students at Level 4 (Stage/Year 4 of the MPharm degree/Masters level) should tackle the tasks through to the end, as should pre-registration students and indeed pharmacists. To differentiate between learning at different stages of study, the following approach is taken. Each learning outcome is preceded by the sentence, 'On successful completion of the cases, Level [1–4] readers will be able to ...'. The outcomes for each stage of learning are then expressed appropriately using suitable verbs and this gives the opportunity to the reader to determine that they have learnt/achieved the outcome at the correct level. A number of learning points are raised by each of the cases. Although readers at any level of learning can attempt all of the set tasks, the task objectives are presented in a level-specific manner so as to ensure the educational objectives are met by students at gradually advancing levels of learning.

For the purpose of this book, students at Level 1 are expected to give evidence of *knowledge*. Verbs that match this level of learning include (Figure 7.1):

- 'describe' (i.e., write down relevant information)
- 'define' (i.e., state the nature or meaning of something)
- 'reproduce' (i.e., produce a copy of something).

Students at Level 2 are expected to give evidence of *comprehension*. Verbs that match this level of learning include:

- 'summarise' (i.e., state only the main features of an argument)
- 'interpret' (i.e., explain the meaning of something)
- 'indicate' (i.e., point something out).

Students in the transition from Level 2 to Level 3 are expected to give evidence of *application of knowledge or understanding*. Verbs that match this level of learning include:

- 'verify' (i.e., to ascertain the correctness of something by a process of examination)
- 'choose' (i.e., pick something out as being most suitable from alternative options)
- 'demonstrate' (i.e., show the truth of something by using evidence or giving proof).

Students at Level 3 are expected to give evidence of *analysis*. Verbs that match this level of learning include:

- 'justify' (i.e., present a valid argument to support a given theory or conclusion)
- 'criticise' (i.e., form and express a judgement about something)
- 'analyse' (i.e., separate the issue into its component parts and show how they interrelate).

Students from Level 4 onwards, are expected to give evidence of *synthesis*. Verbs that match this level of learning include:

- 'formulate' (i.e., create or prepare methodically)
- 'put together' (i.e., assemble from constituent parts)
- 'create' (bring something new into existence).

They should also be able to give evidence of *evaluation*. Verbs that match this level of learning include:

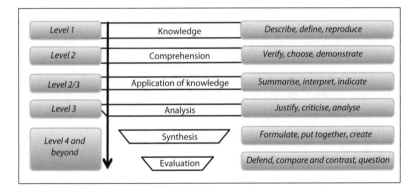

Figure 7.1 An illustration of the progression of learning through the stages of a degree from Level 1 to Level 4 (Masters), and beyond.

- 'defend' (i.e., write in favour or attempt to justify something)
- 'compare and contrast' (i.e., point out the similarities and differences in a logical way)
- 'question' (i.e., express doubt or raise objections about something).

Learning outcomes

The following learning outcomes are anticipated as a result of successfully completing the tasks in relation to the cases outlined in this chapter:

- Level 1 readers will be able to accurately reproduce the facts relevant to the cases.
- Level 2 readers will be able to interpret the cases and indicate pertinent theories.
- Level 2/3 readers will be able to choose the major problems to be resolved.
- Level 3 readers will be able to justify their solutions to the problems identified.
- Level 4 readers will be able to put together a robust recommendation from their own perspective.
- Level 4 readers will be able to defend their recommendation in light of potential criticism.

The cases are arranged as three groups, involving:

- consultations for self-care
- consultations for health promotion
- prescribed medication.

Tasks

The following tasks accompany each case presented in this chapter. You will notice that those at Level 1 of MPharm learning are required only to work through Task 1 in relation to each case, whereas those at Level 2 should work through both Tasks 1 and 2, and so on. The tasks cannot be skipped though – you must work through the logical sequence of the tasks to fully benefit from the learning objectives.

Level 1: establish the basic facts

Use the following questions to help you establish some of the basic facts in each case. Refer to the case scenario and where necessary use quotations or paraphrase to demonstrate your understanding.

- Who are the main characters involved in the case?
- What (if any) is the historical relationship between the main characters?
- What is the flow of events?
- Is there a deadline for reaching a recommendation?

Level 2: identify the problems

Use the following questions to help you identify all the potential problems and issues in the case scenario. You should link each problem to some underlying theory only if possible and of course provide actual evidence from the case.

- What are all the potential questions/problems?
- Which are the factors relevant to the problems?
- What has compounded or even created the problems?
- What issues would normally need further clarification – what do you need to make assumptions about to proceed with the case?

Level 2/3: make a statement about the major issue(s)

Use the following questions to help you make a statement about the major issue(s) in the case. You should link this statement to underlying theory and again provide actual evidence from the case scenario.

- What are your feelings after reading the case?
- What is the main problem as far as each protagonist is concerned?
- What are two or three major issues as far as you are concerned?

Level 3: generate potential solutions

Use the following questions to help you generate as many viable solutions to deal with the major issue(s) in the case, as identified above. Link this statement to underlying theory if possible.

- What are the practical solutions to each of the major issues identified above?
- What can facilitate the solutions?

Level 4: make a robust recommendation

Use the following questions to help you generate a statement of recommendation to deal with the major issue(s) in the case scenario. This can include one or more of the potential solutions identified above. Link this statement to underlying theory, justify the choice and explain how it will solve the major problems. Make sure that your statement of recommendation details a precise course of action.

- What ought to happen?
- What must be done to resolve the situation, by whom, when and in what sequence?

Level 4: reflect on your recommendation

Use the following questions to help you reflect on your recommendation, above. Link your reflections to alternative underlying theory where possible.

- Would all the protagonists be happy with what you have recommended? *And/or:* How would your colleagues criticise your recommendation?
- How would you justify your choice in light of others' assessment?

Concepts to consider

The following is a checklist of concepts to consider as you work through each case – the chapters should be consulted for in-depth information. The concepts relate directly to theory presented in Chapters 1, 3, 4, 5 and 6 inclusive. Concepts from Chapter 2 are considered separately in Chapter 8. You are encouraged to read and consider for yourself the merits and drawbacks of including each concept as part of the analytical process. A sample case has been examined in detail to provide guidance (see 'Worked example') – do make sure you read this in full.

Some dos

Chapter 1:

- Consider social determinants in relation to each case – could the patient's socioeconomic class, gender, education, neighbourhood conditions and communities, lifetime or generational factors, working conditions, income and wealth or race be affecting their health?
- Consider behavioural factors in relation to each case – could risky health behaviours such as smoking, alcohol, diet and exercise be affecting the patient's health?

Chapter 3:

- Consider the impact of heuristics and cognitive biases – are everyday assumptions being made which in turn result in misleading reasoning?
- Consider the impact of people's attributions – who are the characters blaming for events and is their reasoning necessarily sound?
- Consider the impact of people's emotions on their thinking – could the characters' attention, memory and interpretation be influenced by their emotional state?
- Consider the impact of people's thoughts and behaviour on their emotions – could negative thinking be affecting the characters' mood? Is there scope for people to revise their perspective to avoid undue negativity?

Chapter 4:

- Consider the relevance of the health belief model in relation to the case – in what way could the characters' behaviour be captured by the core concepts presented in the model?
- Consider the relevance of the social cognitive theory in relation to the case – in what way could the characters' behaviour be captured by the core concepts presented in the model?
- Consider the relevance of the reasoned action approach in relation to the case – in what way could the characters' behaviour be captured by the core concepts presented in the model?
- Consider the relevance of the transtheoretical model of change in relation to the case – at which stage of change are the characters in relation to their behaviour?
- Consider the relevance of the fuzzy-trace theory in relation to the case – what are people's likely gist representations? How are these being incorporated with their thinking, values and principles?
- Consider what the cognitive models outlined above would recommend for instigating behaviour change – is there any one model you could apply to help you determine the best course of action to take in relation to the case?

Chapter 5:

- Consider the impact of factors that may be affecting adherence to medicines, if relevant – could social and economic factors, healthcare and system-related factors, condition/disease-related factors, therapy-related factors or patient-related factors be influencing adherence?
- Consider how the patient is adjusting to chronic illness, if relevant – are social factors or outlook on life affecting how the patient is coping with their condition?

- Consider the relevance of Lazarus's transactional model of stress in relation to the case, if relevant – in what way could the characters' coping behaviour or experience of stress be explained by their primary or secondary appraisal of the situation according to this model?

- Consider the relevance of Leventhal's common-sense model of self-regulation in relation to the case, if relevant – in what way could the patients' management of their chronic illness be captured by the core concepts presented in the model?

- Consider the relevance of illness representations in relation to the case, if relevant – in what way could the patients' management of their chronic illness be captured by the core concepts presented in the Illness Perception Questionnaire?

- Consider the relevance of the necessity–concerns framework in relation to the case, if relevant – in what way could the patients' management of their treatment regimen be captured by the core concepts presented in the framework?

- Consider interventions for improving adherence to medication, if relevant – is there any one intervention (or more) that you could recommend in relation to the case?

Chapter 6:

- Consider the NICE recommendations for improving adherence to medication, if relevant – how could these be incorporated into your own recommendations about the handling of the case?

- Consider the practitioner–patient relationship in the case – is patient-centred care being practised and what would your recommendations include?

- Consider the appropriateness of shared decision making in the case – are the patient and the practitioner likely to want to become involved in shared decision making and how could this concept be incorporated into your recommendations about the handling of the case?

- Consider the importance of emotional intelligence in relation to the case – are emotions being perceived, understood and managed optimally?

- Consider the body language described in the case – what are the non-verbal signals, for example, eye contact, facial expressions, spatial distance, posture and gesture indicating?

- Consider the usefulness of cultivating body language to enhance the communication within the case – could you recommend particular use of body language to improve rapport?

- Consider the relevance of cognitive appraisals of the situation by the characters involved – are the protagonists making incorrect interpretations that are then influencing their emotions?
- Consider whether the characters' erroneous thoughts could be better managed, if relevant – is there a cognitive restructuring technique you could recommend to help the characters better manage the situation described?

Some don'ts

- Don't attempt to solve all of the problems in the case – after identifying the problems, as you work through the tasks, determine the relevance of the material presented and prioritise the issues.
- At the same time, avoid superficial recommendations or 'quick fixes' that treat only the 'symptoms' of the problem.
- Don't attempt to bring in all of the theory you have learnt as part of the solution – you should use the opportunity to apply (and defend) theory/theories that you consider most robust.
- Don't try to change the world with your answer – it is unlikely you will be able to make a seismic shift in attitudes so tackle issues that can be tackled within the setting.
- Therefore, avoid unrealistic recommendations – make sure your recommendations can be realistically implemented or they are not real solutions.
- Don't blame the scenario if you are unable to answer the question – you have been provided with ample information to enable you to tackle the case.
- Avoid taking sides – provide a non-judgemental and professional answer that does not discriminate against the characters involved.
- Don't waffle or use superfluous words to describe your recommendation – use the SMART acronym if necessary, which states that objectives should be specific, measurable, attainable, relevant and time-bound.
- Don't expect that there will be a perfect answer or that you will be provided with the 'right' answer – the purpose of the case is to make you think widely and ultimately focus in on what you prioritise to be important as a result of your own judgement.

Worked example

The following scenario has been 'deconstructed' first, to illustrate the type of preliminary analysis that might take place as you work through the case studies and the accompanying 'tasks', recommended above.

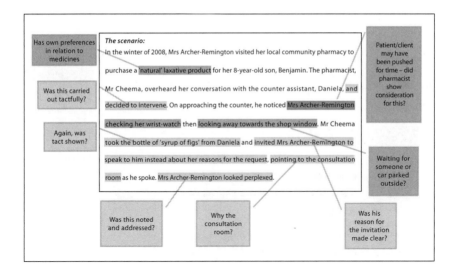

Has own preferences in relation to medicines

Was this carried out tactfully?

Again, was tact shown?

The scenario:
In the winter of 2008, Mrs Archer-Remington visited her local community pharmacy to purchase a 'natural' laxative product for her 8-year-old son, Benjamin. The pharmacist, Mr Cheema, overheard her conversation with the counter assistant, Daniela, and decided to intervene. On approaching the counter, he noticed Mrs Archer-Remington checking her wrist-watch then looking away towards the shop window. Mr Cheema took the bottle of 'syrup of figs' from Daniela and invited Mrs Archer-Remington to speak to him instead about her reasons for the request, pointing to the consultation room as he spoke. Mrs Archer-Remington looked perplexed.

Patient/client may have been pushed for time – did pharmacist show consideration for this?

Waiting for someone or car parked outside?

Was this noted and addressed?

Why the consultation room?

Was his reason for the invitation made clear?

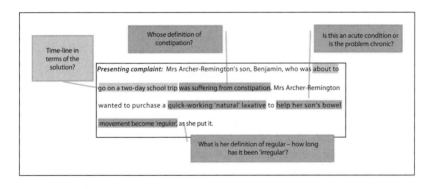

Time-line in terms of the solution?

Whose definition of constipation?

Is this an acute condition or is the problem chronic?

Presenting complaint: Mrs Archer-Remington's son, Benjamin, who was about to go on a two-day school trip was suffering from constipation. Mrs Archer-Remington wanted to purchase a quick-working 'natural' laxative to help her son's bowel movement become 'regular,' as she put it.

What is her definition of regular – how long has it been 'irregular'?

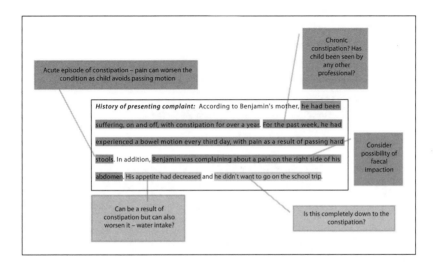

Chronic constipation? Has child been seen by any other professional?

Acute episode of constipation – pain can worsen the condition as child avoids passing motion

History of presenting complaint: According to Benjamin's mother, he had been suffering, on and off, with constipation for over a year. For the past week, he had experienced a bowel motion every third day, with pain as a result of passing hard stools. In addition, Benjamin was complaining about a pain on the right side of his abdomen. His appetite had decreased and he didn't want to go on the school trip.

Consider possibility of faecal impaction

Can be a result of constipation but can also worsen it – water intake?

Is this completely down to the constipation?

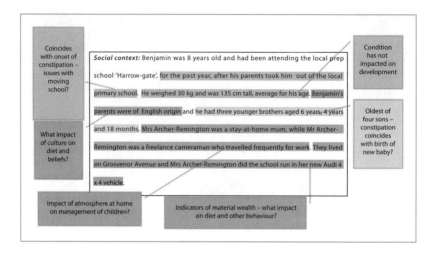

Coincides with onset of constipation – issues with moving school?

What impact of culture on diet and beliefs?

Condition has not impacted on development

Oldest of four sons – constipation coincides with birth of new baby?

Social context: Benjamin was 8 years old and had been attending the local prep school 'Harrow-gate', for the past year, after his parents took him out of the local primary school. He weighed 30 kg and was 135 cm tall, average for his age. Benjamin's parents were of English origin and he had three younger brothers aged 6 years, 4 years and 18 months. Mrs Archer-Remington was a stay-at-home mum, while Mr Archer-Remington was a freelance cameraman who travelled frequently for work. They lived on Grosvenor Avenue and Mrs Archer-Remington did the school run in her new Audi 4 x 4 vehicle.

Impact of atmosphere at home on management of children?

Indicators of material wealth – what impact on diet and other behaviour?

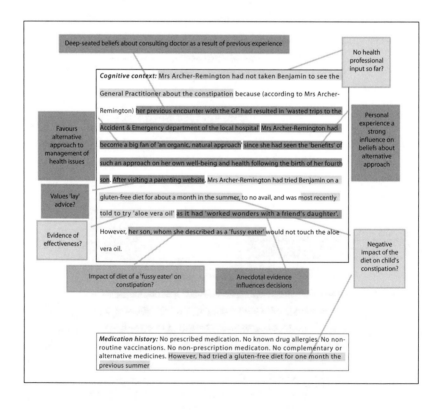

Deep-seated beliefs about consulting doctor as a result of previous experience

No health professional input so far?

Cognitive context: Mrs Archer-Remington had not taken Benjamin to see the General Practitioner about the constipation because (according to Mrs Archer-Remington) her previous encounter with the GP had resulted in 'wasted trips to the Accident & Emergency department of the local hospital' Mrs Archer-Remington had become a big fan of 'an organic, natural approach' since she had seen the 'benefits' of such an approach on her own well-being and health following the birth of her fourth son. After visiting a parenting website, Mrs Archer-Remington had tried Benjamin on a gluten-free diet for about a month in the summer, to no avail, and was most recently told to try 'aloe vera oil' as it had 'worked wonders with a friend's daughter'. However, her son, whom she described as a 'fussy eater' would not touch the aloe vera oil.

Favours alternative approach to management of health issues

Values 'lay' advice?

Evidence of effectiveness?

Personal experience a strong influence on beliefs about alternative approach

Negative impact of the diet on child's constipation?

Impact of diet of a 'fussy eater' on constipation?

Anecdotal evidence influences decisions

Medication history: No prescribed medication. No known drug allergies. No non-routine vaccinations. No non-prescription medicaton. No complementary or alternative medicines. However, had tried a gluten-free diet for one month the previous summer

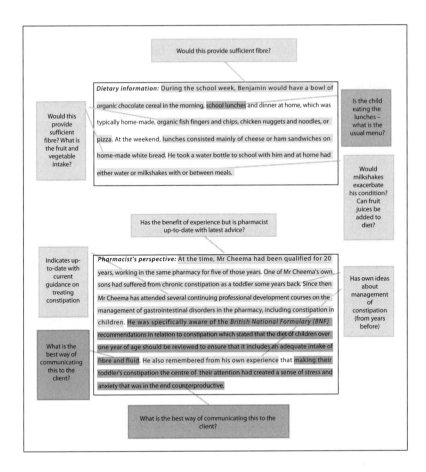

How to tackle the task: Mrs Archer-Remington and Benjamin's constipation

Revisit the generic tasks listed at the beginning of this chapter to complete your learning:

Level 1: establish the basic facts

Use the following questions to help you establish some of the basic facts in this case. Refer to the case scenario and, where necessary, use quotations or paraphrase to demonstrate your understanding.

Who are the main characters involved in this case?

The main characters are Mrs Archer-Remington (the patient's mother), Benjamin Archer-Remington (the patient), Mr Cheema (the pharmacist), and, briefly, Daniela (the counter assistant).

What (if any) is the historical relationship between the main characters?

Mrs Archer-Remington is Benjamin's mother. She is clearly 'in charge' of Benjamin's health and, to some extent, dietary intake of food. She decides how to deal with Benjamin's constipation. Mr Cheema is the pharmacist and although he has been at the same pharmacy for five years, he does not appear to have any particular rapport with Mrs Archer-Remington, who did not ask to see him initially. Daniela is the counter assistant – perhaps she is not yet experienced; nonetheless there does not appear to be mutual respect in the relationship with the pharmacist.

What is the flow of events?

Benjamin Archer-Remington's mother had a new baby over a year ago, which was soon followed by Benjamin himself being moved from the local primary school to a new private school. Around the same time, Benjamin started to show signs of constipation. His diet does not appear to contain sufficient amounts of fibre and fruit and vegetables to ensure regular bowel movements and he may not be receiving the right hydration. Benjamin's mother is keen on a natural approach and tried him on a gluten-free diet, which did not improve the constipation. Around a week ago, he developed an acute episode of constipation which is accompanied by pain on passing a motion and pain on the right side of the abdomen. Benjamin has lost his appetite. He is about to go on a school trip, which he does not wish to attend.

Is there a deadline for reaching a recommendation?

Immediate resolution sought by Mrs Archer-Remington.

Level 2: identify the problems

Use the following questions to help you identify all the potential problems and issues in this case. You should link each problem to some underlying theory only if possible and of course provide actual evidence from the case scenario.

What are the potential questions/problems?

The list includes:

- The chronic, unmanaged constipation (which began a year before, as evidenced in the case).

    Theory: Lazarus's transactional model of stress might be relevant in terms of Benjamin's ability to cope with the constipation as a chronic condition. The inability to cope – for example, if brought on by the change of school environment – might be leading to stress and exacerbation of the condition.

- The acute episode of constipation (onset a week before, as evidenced in the case).

    Theory: Domains of the Illness Perception Questionnaire could be used to conceptualise mother's attitude to the acute episode of constipation: identity, time line, cause, consequence, control.

- Mrs Archer-Remington's approach to solving health problems (on her own admission).

  Theory: Heuristics and cognitive biases influence Mrs Archer-Remington's views about health professionals (consulting with the doctor) and decisions about managing health (her preference for a 'natural' approach).

- The pharmacist's ability to exert influence in the long-run (this is a question rather than a 'problem' – there is no evidence but an inkling from reading the case).

  Theory: The health belief model and its constructs may be useful in terms of whether the pharmacist is able to influence a desired change: seriousness of chronic constipation, susceptibility, cues to action, benefits and barriers to taking action. Emotional intelligence is also important.

You may wish to identify other problems and add them to the above list.

Which are the factors relevant to the problems?

- The child is constipated, in pain, has lost his appetite and does not want to go on the school trip (as described by the mother).

  Theory: Using Lazarus's transactional model of stress may lead one to conclude that the acute episode is feeding back into any stress already experienced by Benjamin as a result of his long-term constipation.

- Mrs Archer-Remington needs a quick solution to the acute constipation because she is expecting her child to go on the school trip (as described by the mother).

  Theory: Using the domains of the Illness Perception Questionnaire to conceptualise the mother's attitude to the acute episode of constipation, one could hypothesise that the mother recognises the episode as acute constipation, with a short time line – i.e., she is expecting it to clear up. It is not clear what she sees as the cause. In terms of the consequence, it could be hypothesised that perhaps she is focused mainly on the child's inability to attend the 'school trip' rather than other consequences such as the pain being experienced by Benjamin. The mother thinks the constipation can be controlled by a 'quick-acting, natural laxative'.

- Mrs Archer-Remington prefers a 'natural' approach to solving health problems (as described by the mother).

  Theory: You could consider the role of the mother's heuristics as part of Leventhal's common-sense model. For the mother, her time–space mapping might mean the condition should be manageable within a short space of time with conventional (albeit 'natural') medication; the pattern of symptoms points to constipation, which although she had previously not considered it to be an urgent problem, is now a real issue that she cannot control but wishes to control. In terms of her cultural beliefs she might be seeing the constipation as a natural part of childhood; certainly, to the mother, other parents appear to have experienced similar issues with their children which they have managed to solve the natural way.

- The pharmacist is up-to-date and keen to help in the short- and long-run but may be lacking the optimal communication skills needed (as demonstrated by his treatment – sidelining – of Daniela, the counter assistant).

  Theory: Is the pharmacist's ability to practise patient-centred care and carry out shared decision making important? Can the pharmacist use emotional intelligence and body language to best effect?

You may wish to identify other problems and add them to the above list.

What has compounded or even created the problems?

- The child's normal diet does not seem conducive to a good bowel habit and he is deemed a 'fussy eater' (assumed from dietary information provided).

  Theory: Returning to the Illness Perception Questionnaire in association with Leventhal's model, does the mother realise that the child's diet could be a cause of the problem?

- The constipation itself may have lowered the child's appetite, which could further affect his diet (assumed from information provided).

  Theory: See comments, immediately above.

- Trial-and-error with alternative approaches rather than involvement of health professionals has resulted in constipation that is not currently 'managed' with any health professional involvement (assumed from information provided).

  Theory: A number of issues exist in relation to the mother's perception of health professionals, as well as the management of constipation. This could be related to power sharing in the patient–doctor relationship; there have been previous occasions where the paternalistic approach of the doctor did not suit the mother's preferences for involvement in decisions. The mother is currently showing a preference for the 'consumerist' approach by asking to buy a quick-acting natural laxative from the pharmacy.

- There may be underlying psychological factors associated with the constipation: the birth of a new baby at home, Benjamin being the oldest of four sons, and moving to a new school – perhaps the child doesn't like visiting the toilet at the new school? Or perhaps he doesn't like the new school – he certainly does not want to attend the school trip (assumed from information provided).

Theory: Returning to Lazarus's transactional model of stress may lead one to conclude that Benjamin needs to be empowered to feel he can regain control of his condition to reduce the stress he might be experiencing.

You may wish to identify other problems and add them to the above list.

Which issues would normally need further clarification? Which assumptions do you need to make to proceed with the case?

- The school menu and whether the child is actually eating the food on offer (unclear from the information provided).

  Theory: See comment about the cause of the illness.

- The child's own interpretation of the causes of his constipation and why it is worsening are not yet established – assumptions are being made about the child's relationship with the school (unclear from the information provided).

  Theory: See interpretations being made using Lazarus's model.

- Does the child take sufficient exercise?

  Theory: Could this be a potential factor in terms of the cause of the illness.

You may wish to identify other problems and add them to the above list.

Level 2/3: make a statement about the major issue(s)

Use the following questions to help you make a statement about the major issue(s) in this case. You should link this statement to underlying theory and again provide actual evidence from the case.

What are your feelings after reading the case?

- The mother has quite a different understanding of the problem and priority, in terms of solving the problem, compared with the pharmacist, and it might be quite difficult to exert great influence in one consultation.

  Theory: The application of emotional intelligence would be vital in this case.

You may wish to identify other problems and add them to the above list.

What is the main problem as far as each protagonist is concerned?

- A natural approach to curing her child's acute constipation appears to be Mrs Archer-Remington's primary concern (as she states about wanting a quick-acting, natural laxative).

Theory: See comments above, but in summary and in relation to the control of her son's issue, it appears the mother believes that she can ask for a quick-acting natural laxative and that will solve the problem.

- The impending school trip appears to be Benjamin's primary concern (as Mrs Archer-Remington relays).

  Theory: See comments above but, in summary, the pain and potential issues relating to school mean that Benjamin does not want the added pressure of having to attend the school trip while constipated.

- The overall management of the child's constipation is Mr Cheema's primary concern (as evidenced in the case).

  Theory: See comments above but, in summary, the pharmacist probably wants to resolve the overall problem with constipation, looking at root causes and options for resolving the condition permanently.

You may wish to identify alternative suggestions to those listed above.

What are two or three major issues as far as you are concerned?

- Managing the acute constipation for now.

  Theory: Using emotional intelligence and the other theories applied to the case should be a priority, to persuade the mother to act in Benjamin's best interests in terms of the acute episode, which may have to involve a visit to the doctor.

- Attempting to manage the chronic constipation in the long term.

  Theory: Using emotional intelligence and the other theories applied to the case, to persuade the mother to consider long-term behavioural changes to resolve the issue.

You may wish to identify alternative issues to those listed above.

Level 3: generate potential solutions

Use the following questions to help you generate as many viable solutions to deal with the major issue(s) in this case, as identified above. Link this statement to underlying theory if possible.

What are the practical solutions to each of the major issues identified above?

- Managing the acute constipation for now

  o Keeping the child off school until the condition is managed.

     Theory: See comments in relation to Lazarus's model and Leventhal's model.

o Recommending a laxative that will help bowel movement.

Theory: See comments in relation to mother's preferred model of interaction with health professionals (consumerist).

o Adding any fruit or vegetables to the diet that the child will tolerate and ensuring adequate intake of water – cutting out food known to be counterproductive.

Theory: See above in relation to cause and control of the condition.

o Monitoring the pain and recommending a medical examination if no improvement is seen in the next 24 hours, or sooner if the pain worsens.

Theory: See above in relation to control of the condition.

o Avoiding overt focus on the child's constipation in front of him.

Theory: See comments in relation to Lazarus's model.

You may wish to identify alternative/additional issues to those listed above.

- Attempting to manage the chronic constipation in the long-run

    o Reviewing the patient again in a week's time.

    Theory: Emotional intelligence would dictate now is not the time to start 'lecturing' the mother about long-term changes. This would be better conducted once a trusting relationship has been established.

    o Proposing a conversation about changes that can be made to ensure resolution of the chronic problem.

    Theory: As above.

You may wish to identify alternative/additional issues to those listed above.

What can facilitate the solutions?

- A non-judgemental approach.

    Theory: Using emotional intelligence and body language skills.

- Packaging the information in a way that Mrs Archer-Remington will take up.

    Theory: Using the theories outlined above to appeal to Mrs Archer-Remington's preferences for information. For example: appealing to her need for a quick solution by providing a product as requested (consumerist expectation); matching her reliance on anecdotal information and heuristic reasoning by quoting examples of other people with similar experiences, in a way that introduces Mrs Archer-Remington to the idea that perhaps the consequences are deeper than she has considered (e.g., effect on psychological health of child with constipation).

- Avoiding being over-ambitious.

Theory: Using emotional intelligence and body language skills with the primary aim of building rapport rather than attempting to solve all the problems at once.

- Use of good communication skills.

Theory: Using emotional intelligence and body language skills.

You may wish to identify alternative/additional ideas to those listed above.

Level 4: make a robust recommendation

Use the following questions to help you generate a statement of recommendation to deal with the major issue(s) in this case. This can include one or more of the potential solutions identified above. Link this statement to underlying theory, justify the choice and explain how it will solve the major problems. Make sure that your statement of recommendation details a precise course of action.

What ought to happen?

- Treating the child's acute constipation must be prioritised over and above any other consideration because the child is distraught and has lost his appetite, which could worsen his condition further.

What must be done to resolve the situation, by whom, when and in what sequence?

- The pharmacist should use language that will appeal to the patient's mother to encourage her to keep the child off school while the acute episode of constipation is brought under control – this could mean the child would be missing out on the school trip but the trip is not the priority here. To appeal to the mother's preference for heuristic-based decision making, to bring the acute condition under control, the pharmacist could use an anecdotal example to highlight similar cases where the approach being recommended has been successful, stating the benefits to the child.

Theory: Leventhal's common-sense model of self-regulation and health belief model.

- The pharmacist can recommend a laxative for now with the explicit advice that medical advice is sought within 24 hours if the condition does not improve or sooner if the pain worsens. This is to appeal to the mother's apparent preference for a consumerist approach to the problem.

Theory: Power-sharing in the patient–professional relationship.

- The pharmacist can offer to see the patient's mother again when she is ready, to provide advice that can help solve the chronic constipation. This is in an attempt to build a rapport with the mother and to slowly devise a plan that she might use at a time when she is ready.

Theory: Emotional intelligence and effective use of body language.

Level 4: reflect on your recommendation

Use the following questions to help you reflect on your recommendation, above. Link your reflections to alternative underlying theory where possible.

Would all the protagonists be happy with what you have recommended? And/or: How would your colleagues criticise your recommendation?

- Colleagues might criticise the approach because it 'gives in' to the mother's preference for a product from the pharmacy.
- Some may also suggest that the patient be sent to the general practitioner as a matter of urgency.
- Others may also criticise the approach for not attempting to address the chronic condition there and then in the one consultation.

You may wish to identify alternative/additional criticisms to those listed above.

How would you justify your choice in light of others' assessment?

- Selling a pharmacy product suitable for constipation in an 8-year-old is unlikely to do any harm and may even help, with the proviso that medical attention is sought after 24 hours and earlier if symptoms worsen.
- Gaining the client's trust is more important and any health message given is more likely to be taken up at a time when they are ready to make changes – not at a time that suits the health professional and their need for information provision.

Additional suggested student assignments

Although readers are encouraged to work through the tasks above as part of their independent learning, teachers at university may also wish to incorporate some of the cases and tasks as part of formal courses. In that case, the suggestions listed below may prove useful.

Workshops

The cases can be used within formal workshops. Students could be asked to read them beforehand. During the workshop and in their groups, students could be asked to engage in role play to portray the salient points from each case. After working through the 'tasks' outlined above, students could be asked to engage in a second role play exercise to act out their recommendations. Alternatively, or in combination, student groups could be asked to present their thoughts and recommendations using acetate slides or flipchart posters prepared as group work in class.

Posters

The cases could be used as part of formal assessment of learning. Students in groups could be assigned a case and given prior notice to work together to prepare a printed poster to match the 'tasks' outlined above. Posters and accompanying student presentations, usually at Level 3 or 4 of the MPharm course, could then be assessed formally using a template such as that presented in the box.

Suggested template for marking poster presentations of the cases

Scoring each component of the marking criteria

0 Clear fail. No evidence of these criteria having been addressed.

1 Clear fail. It is possible to acknowledge that some attempt has been made to address these criteria, but this has been completely unsuccessful.

2 Clear fail. It is possible to acknowledge that some attempt has been made to address these criteria, but this has been largely unsuccessful.

3 Inadequate work. Some of the work showing evidence of these criteria having been met, but insufficient to merit a pass grade.

4 Bare pass. There is evidence that these criteria have been met.

5 Adequate work. It is clear that these criteria have been met.

6 Good work. In respect of these criteria, the work represents a good, solid performance at Masters' level.

7 Very good work. In respect of these criteria, the work represents a very good performance at Masters' level.

8 Very strong work. In respect of these criteria, the work represents a strong performance at Masters' level.

9 Distinction. In respect of these criteria, the work represents an excellent performance at Masters' level.

10 Clear distinction. The work is outstanding in meeting these criteria at Masters' level.

Marking criteria for verbal delivery:
(40% – can be varied to suit academic setting)

• overall coherence as a group

• eye contact with the audience

- voice projection
- visual impact of poster
- clarity of poster content.

Marking criteria for content of presentation:
(60% – can be varied to suit academic setting)
- establish the basic facts
- identify the problems
- making a statement about the major issue(s)
- generating potential solutions
- making a robust recommendation
- reflecting on the recommendation.

Presentations

As an alternative to poster presentations, students working in groups could be asked instead to make Microsoft PowerPoint presentations. These could then be assessed formally using a modification of the template presented in the box.

Essays

Students could be asked to work through the cases and to prepare an essay in relation to the 'tasks' outlined above. Word limits could be imposed to match expectations consistent with the stage of learning.

Cases involving consultations for self-care

Ms Walters and constant fatigue

The scenario: Ms Walters normally rushed past the community pharmacy near the city-centre underground station, where she worked. One morning in early spring she went into the pharmacy to buy some tights as she had felt really cold during the journey. She remembered buying a pharmacy-only vitamin capsule some years back from the local pharmacy near her home and decided to enquire about it when she reached the counter. Miss Kallow, the pharmacist, was serving at the counter and came forward to help the gaunt-looking, sallow customer. After observing the patient search the over-the-counter shelving area for a few minutes, Miss Kallow proceeded to ask Ms Walters some general questions to establish what she was after. Ms Walters dismissed her attempts and asked instead for her tights to be put through the till, checking her phone messages several times as she pulled out her purse.

Presenting complaint: Ms Walters had been feeling particularly tired all through winter and didn't want to be struck by yet another cold or flu bug. On a chance visit to the pharmacy, she wanted to purchase a 'strong' vitamin supplement to boost her state of health.

History of presenting complaint: Ms Walters was feeling weary. She had suffered with cold and flu viruses for what seemed to her like months on end. During the morning commute into work that day, she felt particularly chilly and fatigued. Despite her tiredness, Ms Walters found it hard to eat breakfast most mornings. She had a suspected ulcer and 'wanted the (prescribed) capsules to work' before eating anything for the day.

Social context: Ms Walters was 35 years old and worked for a large investment bank in the business district of London. She weighed 50 kg and was 168 cm tall, which made her 'underweight', with a BMI of 17.7. Ms Walters was of mixed English/Spanish origin and lived on her own in the suburbs of west London. She had qualified as an accountant but had since changed fields and now worked as a software manager for one of the city's most coveted companies. Her current job involved managing 17 other staff and saw her working long hours in the week and sometimes at weekends. She rarely found time to go out for leisure activities.

Cognitive context: Ms Walters had visited her local community pharmacy in recent months to have her prescription for omeprazole dispensed and before that to buy cold and flu products. That pharmacist had seemed quite knowledgeable and this encouraged her to seek some advice on her current visit to the city-centre pharmacist. She had suffered from either a sore throat and a stuffy nose or a cough and a fever 'during most of the winter months' but had hoped that the beginning of spring would mark the end of those frequent episodes. To make matters worse, her stomach had begun to 'act up' during that time, which the doctor had described as a suspected ulcer. She had been told to take a four-week course of an anti-ulcer medicine (omeprazole), which had then been extended to another four weeks. Ms Walters was sure that feeling cold was the first sign of yet another episode of cold or flu and wanted to prevent it by buying some tights to wear on her way to work. She also recalled having taken a 'strong' vitamin supplement some years ago, which she could only buy from the pharmacy.

Medication history: At the time, she had been taking omeprazole capsules 20 mg daily for a suspected gastric ulcer for seven weeks. No known drug allergies. No non-routine vaccinations. No current non-prescription medication but she had been taking over-the-counter products for colds and flu during the winter months. No complementary or alternative medicines but she had taken a pharmacy-only vitamin supplement some 15 years earlier.

Dietary information: Ms Walters often skipped breakfast, but had a coffee and a small biscuit about mid-morning. Lunch was normally a sandwich and a fizzy drink with dinner a ready-meal warmed up in the microwave or some noodles and vegetables stir-fried on the hob. Ms Walters didn't shop at weekends, preferring to visit the local supermarket on returning home after work when needed. Meals at the weekend were normally an attempt to use up whatever was left in the fridge or the cupboard.

Pharmacist's perspective: Miss Kallow had qualified the previous summer and was working in a different pharmacy from where she had trained. A bright and chirpy character, she was eager to please and prove herself a worthy pharmacist. Although she believed she had received very good training, she didn't recall having come across a pharmacy-only vitamin supplement. She really wanted to help Ms Walters though, as she judged her to be particularly 'ill-looking'. She thought that a good approach would be to instigate the WWHAM questioning routine, which is made up of questions about *w*ho the medicine is for, *w*hat the symptoms are, *h*ow long they have been ill, *a*ction taken so far, and *m*edicines being taken at the moment. However, this line of questioning seemed particularly futile with Ms Walters and when she started to terminate the line of questioning, Miss Kallow panicked and thought of all sorts of serious illnesses she might be missing by failing to engage with Ms Walters.

Mr Smithers and back pain

The scenario: Mr Smithers was often seen on a Saturday morning slowly making his way around the supermarket where Miss Khalid was working as a locum pharmacist. Mid-morning one Saturday in January, Mr Smithers approached the counter to ask for a really strong painkiller and perhaps a spray to help relieve his backache. He leaned forward on the counter to relieve the pressure on his back. Miss Khalid, the pharmacist, was called to help the customer, whom she judged immediately as overweight and scruffy, if not 'obese and grubby'. Having looked Mr Smithers up and down briefly, Miss Khalid reached over for a packet of paracetamol and codeine tablets and told Mr Smithers that he could pick up a small tube of diclofenac gel from the shelf unit behind him. She then left the counter assistant to put the tablets through the till, turning away so as to return to the dispensary. Mr Smithers was a little shocked by the lack of attention he had just received.

Presenting complaint: Mr Smithers had a constant pain in his lower back. He wanted to purchase painkiller tablets and perhaps a spray for more immediate relief.

History of presenting complaint: Mr Smithers was continuing with his usual Saturday morning routine despite an unbearable pain in his lower back. He was feeling the 'strain of the post-Christmas month', as he put it. He had taken up a new diet to try and shed the extra weight he had gained during the holidays. The diet seemed to coincide with the back pain.

Social context: Mr Smithers was 52 years old and worked in a DIY shop part-time. He weighed 125 kg and was 196 cm tall, which made him 'obese' with a BMI of 32. Mr Smithers was of English and Welsh origin and lived with his mother in a small flat on the ninth floor of a local, council-owned building. He spent most of his time looking after his mother, who had Parkinson's disease. During the week and on Saturday mornings, his sister would come over to help look after their mother and this enabled Mr Smithers to attend work and do the weekly shopping. As a younger man, Mr Smithers had enjoyed a short stint as a rugby player for a local Welsh team.

Cognitive context: Mr Smithers judged himself to be a relatively content man most of the time, despite the ups and downs he had experienced in his life. His job at the local DIY store kept him in contact with the world of work, and he enjoyed the relief it provided from looking after his mother in the flat. At Christmas, as usual, Mr Smithers had prepared all the meals and this year they had even had a number of visitors come and stay to keep them company. After the festivities, Mr Smithers had found himself a little more breathless than normal and somewhat disappointed because, despite all his good intentions, he had managed to gain yet another 5 kg over the holidays. He had promised his doctor in autumn that he would lose some weight by the New Year. Having seen a programme on television, he had decided to try a drastic new diet on his own. Only a week after the start of the diet, he now found himself with unbearable backache and thought it would be good to ask the pharmacy for some advice. He also had fewer bowel movements than normal, which he put down to the diet.

Medication history: At the time, Mr Smithers had been using one puff of a beclometasone 50 µg inhaler twice daily for mild asthma. He also had a salbutamol inhaler which he had begun to use every other day because of the increased breathlessness. No known drug allergies. No non-routine vaccinations. No current non-prescription medication. No complementary or alternative medicines.

Dietary information: Mr Smithers normally ate a carbohydrate and fat-rich diet and made sure there was a hot dinner of meat and vegetables on the table for him and his mother most nights. He took sandwiches, crisps and chocolates to work normally and on the odd occasion visited the pub after work for a quiet pint with his work mates. His recent diet saw him eating less frequently, which the television programme had advised but he found the cravings unbearable so he was 'topping up' with various sweets.

Pharmacist's perspective: Miss Khalid had accepted that particular locum contract without knowing much about the area. Having found it difficult to obtain a permanent post after her pre-registration training, Miss Khalid was accepting locum contracts where and when she could. Having arrived at the pharmacy that morning, she realised that the dispensing software programme was slightly different from the ones she had used before. Although the dispensing was slow, she had nonetheless found it difficult to keep up with the pace of the pharmacy. She didn't really need the distraction of a simple painkiller request, as she saw it, while she was trying to do her job. She thought that perhaps the counter staff were purposely trying to slow her down when they called her to the counter. When she came to the front, she found Mr Smithers's presence somewhat intimidating and decided to prioritise by making a quick recommendation so that she could get back to the dispensing.

Mr Binty and insomnia

The scenario: Mr Binty was desperately tired. He stopped briefly outside a 24-hour pharmacy to obtain some 'sleeping tablets'. He was about to finish his night-time shift with the mini-cab company in half an hour and was anxious that he would again fail to get to sleep on returning home. The pharmacist was taking a short break and the counter assistant recommended a herbal remedy, which Mr Binty could pick up from the shop floor. Although he would normally try anything and, particularly, natural herbal remedies, Mr Binty felt he really needed something strong that was guaranteed to work. He waited for the pharmacist. In the meantime, he thought about that month's mortgage payment and whether he would still be able to support his sons, both attending university at the time. Mr Binty waited patiently near the counter, his hands overlapping in front of him, looking towards the floor. The pharmacist, Mr Gupta, returned and smiled at the pleasant-looking customer. When he recommended an antihistamine-based product, Mr Gupta was surprised to find that Mr Binty was already taking the same tablets, bought on a previous occasion.

Presenting complaint: Mr Binty was suffering from lack of sleep. He wanted to guarantee a good sleep while at home so that he could concentrate on his driving while at work. Although he had been taking what he believed was a natural product to help him get to sleep, he now wanted something stronger and medicinal from the pharmacist.

History of presenting complaint: Mr Binty had been feeling tired and exhausted. He was working the night shift this week and although he had difficulty getting to sleep when he returned home, his days had become marred by such fatigue that he had even found himself nearly falling asleep while waiting to pick up passengers. He had tried some tablets his wife had recommended at home but they didn't seem to work at all.

Social context: Mr Binty was 60 years old and had worked for the same local mini-cab company for over 15 years. He weighed 75 kg and was 172 cm tall, which made him just 'overweight' with a BMI of 25.4. Mr Binty was of Pakistani origin and lived with his wife and young daughter in a small house on Hatton Terrace. His second child had this month started university, which meant that he was now expected to support both sons in their efforts to study medicine and law. His job involved driving for 10 hours a day and he had recently taken the night shift in an attempt to increase his rate of pay. This meant he was working from 7 pm to 5 am, six days a week. He rarely had time to see his daughter, who was starting her GCSEs this year.

Cognitive context: Mr Binty found his mind wondering on to all sorts of subjects, including his financial situation, as soon as he tried to get some sleep at home. He had tried taking some tablets his wife had given him but found that these did not work at all. He was getting more and more tired and this had put a strain on things at home. He certainly didn't want to start worrying his wife too about the finances, as she was, in his opinion, busy enough with the housework and looking after their daughter in the day. He was sure that a tablet from the pharmacy would be strong enough to help him sleep and that one or two days of 'normal' sleep would put him back on the right track. He blamed the lack of sleep on his age because the last time he had tried working nights he had had no trouble at all adjusting within two days.

Medication history: No prescribed medication. No known drug allergies. No non-routine vaccinations. He had been taking an over-the-counter anti-histamine product for insomnia for a week believing it to be a herbal remedy. No complementary or alternative medicines.

Dietary information: Mr Binty was taking dinner at home before attending his shift in the evening. Dinner was usually a meat-based spicy dish served with either bread or rice. While at work and to help him keep alert, he had started to have three-hourly cups of coffee in between picking up passengers. After his shift, when he got home in the early hours of the morning, Mr Binty would have a breakfast of bread, jam and tea before retiring to his room. He would then rise at midday for a potato- or samosa-based lunch with his wife.

Pharmacist's perspective: Mr Gupta was an experienced man. He too was in his sixties and he recognised Mr Binty as a pleasant, local man. He thought that Mr Binty looked tired on this occasion. He tried to establish eye contact with the customer, lowering his posture slightly and asked if perhaps Mr Binty wanted to sit and talk in the consultation room. When Mr Binty kindly declined the offer, Mr Gupta then recommended an antihistamine-based product, and found to his surprise that Mr Binty had been taking the very same product for the past week. He recommended Mr Binty come back when he had a little more time but Mr Binty declined, explaining his current work situation. When he realised that the client was in fact working as a mini-cab driver, Mr Gupta experienced a sinking feeling in the pit of his stomach – it was not wise to recommend an antihistamine product, as he just had, to someone whose job it was to keep alert and drive at night.

Mrs Kermani-Zartosht and antimalarial tablets

The scenario: In the spring of 2005, Mrs Kermani-Zartosht was frantically preparing for an exciting holiday home, to Iran. She visited the pharmacy on her daughter's request to find out if her daughter and son-in-law, who would both be travelling with her for the first time, would need antimalarial tablets for the trip. The counter assistant, Jenny, asked how many people were travelling with Mrs Kermani-Zartosht, which regions they were travelling to and how long they were staying. After checking the risk of malaria, Jenny recommended three travel packs, each containing 98 tablets of proguanil (100 mg) and 14 tablets of chloroquine (250 mg). She proceeded to explain the dosing schedule, speaking loudly and clearly. Mrs Kermani-Zartosht started frowning and muttering quietly under her breath before accusing the counter assistant of insulting her intelligence. She asked to speak to the manager straightaway.

Presenting complaint: Mrs Kermani-Zartosht was travelling to a high-risk malaria region with her daughter and son-in-law. She had been sent to the pharmacy to find out if her daughter and son-in-law needed antimalarial tablets for the trip.

History of presenting complaint: Mrs Kermani-Zartosht visited her home country every two years. She normally stayed in Tehran, a vast and modern city. This time she was taking her daughter and son-in-law with her on what she believed would be an exciting tour of the southern region of the country, her own birthplace. Her daughter had not been back to Iran since the age of five and Mrs Kermani-Zartosht's son-in-law had never visited the country.

Social context: Mrs Kermani-Zartosht was 65 years old and although long retired, had held a management post at a bank in Tehran some 25 years back. She weighed 73 kg and was 162 cm tall, which made her 'overweight' with a BMI of 27.8. Mrs Kermani-Zartosht was of Iranian origin and lived with her two cats on the ground floor of an apartment block by the river in London's Chelsea region. Her husband, who had died some 10 years back, had been a businessman and before that, in Iran, a general in the previous administration's army. Her daughter and son-in-law were busy accountants working for separate firms in the City. Mrs Kermani-Zartosht had a wide circle of friends and often held dinner parties at her home, entertaining some very elite guests at times.

Cognitive context: Mrs Kermani-Zartosht had been to Iran dozens of times and had never taken antimalarial tablets, which she thought might be needed by 'foreigners' after her daughter had persuaded her to check the requirements. It was the first time her daughter and son-in-law were visiting the country with her, and she wanted 'everything to be perfect'. Her son-in-law, who had travelled extensively in his gap-year and since then on company business, was used to taking antimalarial tablets and was under the impression that southern Iran fell into the malaria zone. On hearing the counter assistant's tone, Mrs Kermani-Zartosht judged her as being 'patronising' and became suspicious that she was being treated as someone with very little intelligence. In any case, she experienced some trouble deciphering the dosing information being relayed to her by the counter assistant, whom she also judged was trying to sell her one too many packs of tablets. As far as Mrs Kermani-Zartosht was concerned, if there was any malaria in Bam, she had immunity to it as she was born and brought up in that region.

Medication history: Mrs Kermani-Zartosht was taking celecoxib 100 mg tablets in two divided doses for osteoarthritis in her knee. No known drug allergies. No non-routine vaccinations. No current non-prescription medication. No complementary or alternative medicines. Her daughter and son-in-law had no recent medication history.

Dietary information: Mrs Kermani-Zartosht enjoyed a breakfast of freshly brewed jasmine and Darjeeling tea, breads, conserves and cheeses. Lunch was normally a rice-based dish, unless she was preparing for a dinner party, in which case she skipped lunch. Her dinner parties were well known for the rich dishes she made using traditional Iranian recipes. Her shopping was delivered by a friend most weeks.

Pharmacist's perspective: The pharmacist, Mrs Stratton, was called to speak to Mrs Kermani-Zartosht after she had requested to speak to the manager. Mrs Stratton, a middle-aged and experienced hospital pharmacist, was working as the locum pharmacist to help out a friend who was the owner-pharmacist. Mrs Kermani-Zartosht had an assertive presence, which did not threaten Mrs Stratton. The shop was quiet and she was happy to spend the time needed to resolve the situation that had apparently been created by the counter assistant. In Mrs Stratton's opinion, Mrs Kermani-Zartosht had had difficulty understanding the verbal instructions being conveyed by Jenny, the counter assistant. In addition, Mrs Kermani-Zartosht seemed to believe that she was immune to malaria as she had been born in the high-risk malaria region being visited. Mrs Stratton believed it was just a matter of explaining the facts in a way that Mrs Kermani-Zartosht would appreciate.

Ms Pawlowski and earache

The scenario: Ms Ivona Pawlowski often visited her local pharmacy for advice on various aches and pains. She had had problems with her ears for some time and after seeing an advert for a preparation that would help remove ear wax, she had tried the product for several days. At the time, the pharmacist Mr Gresham had taken great care to go through the instructions for use with Ms Pawlowski, using the patient information leaflet as a basis for the conversation. Two weeks later, Ms Pawlowski had returned to the pharmacy with a prescription for betahistine 16 mg tablets, to be taken three times a day. She had asked if she could sit down and wait for the prescription to be made up, because she was feeling particularly unsteady on her feet and couldn't bear to go home and come back again to pick up the medication. On seeing the prescription Mr Gresham was mortified to think that Ms Pawlowski had Ménière's disease, whereas he had sold her a product for removing ear wax just a few weeks earlier.

Presenting complaint: Ms Pawlowski had been experiencing earache for over six months. After trying an over-the-counter wax-removal product for a few days, her daughter had encouraged her to visit a friend who was an ear, nose and throat consultant. He in turn had diagnosed Ms Pawlowski with Ménière's disease.

History of presenting complaint: After having had earache and some loss of hearing, Ms Pawlowski had at first visited the pharmacy and purchased a product for the removal of ear wax. Ms Pawlowski's daughter, Ania, had noticed the product at home and enquired about it. In fact, after a few days of using the product, Ms Pawlowski had also started to experience dizzy spells and some nausea. On hearing this, her daughter Ania had become quite distraught – Ms Pawlowski's mother (Ania's maternal grandmother) had experienced the same symptoms before being diagnosed with a fatal brain tumour some 30 years back. Ania, who was herself a nurse, had urged her mother to visit an ENT specialist, whom she knew through work.

Social context: Ms Pawlowski was 78 years old. She weighed 60 kg and was 168 cm tall, which gave her a BMI of 21 and meant her weight was average. Ms Pawlowski was of eastern European origin and had immigrated to the UK around 50 years earlier with her then husband. They had bought her current house on arrival in the UK with the money she had inherited from her father. The house was in a leafy suburb of London where Ms Pawlowski's daughter, a nurse at the local general hospital, also lived. In her earlier years, Ms Pawlowski had worked as a typist and then secretary before her eyesight had deteriorated in her mid-fifties.

Cognitive context: Ms Pawlowski's father had been a pioneering doctor in Poland, before the war. Although they had stayed in Poland throughout the war and afterwards, Ms Pawlowski and her new husband left for England on her father's death, to build a new life with the money she had inherited from him. This had left the late Mrs Agata Pawlowski (Ms Pawlowski's mother) alone in Poland, where she had developed a fatal brain tumour that had led to her rapid decline and eventual death. Ania had heard the story on many occasions and was anxious to make sure she looked out for similar symptoms in her own mother. In fact, this tragic story had inspired Ania to enter nursing as a profession. Ms Pawlowski did not share her daughter's worries and in fact did not normally disclose her medical problems to her, choosing instead to visit the local pharmacy for health advice.

Medication history: Betaxolol 0.5% eye drops, twice daily for treatment of chronic, simple glaucoma. No known drug allergies. No non-routine vaccinations. She had been using an over-the-counter product containing urea hydrogen peroxide 5% for removal of ear wax in the past two weeks. She had also used various over-the-counter analgesics (tablets and topical products) over the years. No complementary or alternative medicines.

Dietary information: Ms Pawlowski's diet was based on chicken, pork and potatoes with soups in colder weather. She was still able to cook for herself and her daughter and took great pleasure in doing so. Ania did the shopping mainly from local grocers. They took breakfast and dinner together most days while Ms Pawlowski had sandwiches on her own for lunch.

Pharmacist's perspective: Mr Gresham was always pleased to see Ms Pawlowski, a pleasant old lady who seemed to enjoy spending time in his pharmacy. He regularly dispensed her prescription for eye drops and had been only too happy to go through the instructions for the ear drops when she had visited to complain of a blocked, painful ear the previous fortnight. Now he found himself having potentially sold Ms Pawlowski a product that was neither needed nor helpful to her condition. He knew that Ménière's disease was not fatal but at the same time he realised that dizziness, as experienced by most patients with the condition, was not ideal in a frail-looking, elderly lady. He dispensed the betahistine tablets and gave the dispensed item to his counter assistant to hand out to Ms Pawlowski.

Cases involving consultations for health promotion

John and his health behaviours

The scenario: John was reluctant to seek help. He rarely visited the doctor, let alone a pharmacist. Yet his new girlfriend Fiona had taken him to a pharmacy that was running a weight management service. Somewhat embarrassed and at first reluctant to speak to the pharmacist, John admitted that perhaps he would at least like to find out about the programme being offered now that he had made the effort to visit the pharmacy. Patrick, the pharmacist, explained the basis of the weight management service he was offering. It involved taking home a short DVD to watch, and a 30-minute consultation back at the pharmacy after which John could start purchasing his food substitutes on a weekly basis. John was astonished to learn about the cost of the diet.

Presenting complaint: John was brought in by his new girlfriend Fiona to seek advice about losing weight. He had thought that perhaps it was worth looking into this, since he was no longer able to wear his favourite clothes.

History of presenting complaint: John had started dating Fiona, a receptionist at his workplace, about four weeks before. He felt he had to change some of his normal habits if he was going to make the new relationship work. One thing that really did bother John was the extra weight he had been putting on around his stomach, which he associated with a fast-food habit and a generally high-fat diet he had been following for many years. When Fiona recommended a visit to the local pharmacy, John decided to give it a try to keep her happy.

Social context: John was a 42-year-old man of English origin. He weighed 95 kg and was 183 cm tall, with a BMI of 28.4 making him 'overweight' for his age. He worked in an office and had been smoking around 20 cigarettes a day since the age of 15. He socialised with his friends most nights and exceeded the maximum recommended intake of alcohol every Friday and Saturday night. He played pool with a group of colleagues on these nights and it was quite normal for John and his friends to end their evening with a visit to a fast-food outlet in the early hours of Saturday and Sunday mornings. He lived on Rood Lane in a two-bedroom flat that he had rented for the past three years.

Cognitive context: John had first noticed his physique changing when he realised he could no longer buy his clothes from his favourite shop as the sizes didn't fit him any more – but he had ignored the issue for years. On one of the rare nights in with Fiona, they watched a programme called *You Are What You Eat* and John was horrified to see the effect of body fat on the heart and started to think that he should do something about losing weight. He thought that perhaps he could have a go at changing his diet. Fiona had pointed out his other habits too. But he needed his cigarettes to cope with the stressful job. Fiona was 'stressing him out' about this, saying that his yellowing teeth and constant cough were likely to be caused by the smoking. John wondered about a visit to the dentist as a quick solution. The alcohol 'problem', as Fiona called it, was not really a problem to John as he didn't see how it could harm him. All of his friends had been drinking just as much as he had, if not more, and they didn't seem at all concerned. John had never tried a diet before but perhaps Fiona could help him. She was certainly supportive.

Medication history: No prescribed medication. No known drug allergies. No non-routine vaccinations. No non-prescription medication. No complementary or alternative medicines.

Dietary information: During the working week, John would have bacon sandwiches and coffee for breakfast, sandwiches for lunch and a ready-meal for dinner. At the weekend, dinner was around 10 units of alcohol followed by kebabs and chips in the early hours of Saturday and Sunday mornings. Most evenings if he went out after work, he had at least one pint of lager, if not two, before returning to have dinner alone. His routine had changed a little with Fiona but his diet was almost the same.

Pharmacist's perspective: At the time, Patrick had been promoting a commercial weight-loss programme for six months. It was the first commercially viable programme that Patrick had encountered and he was very keen to promote its uptake in his pharmacy. The programme did appear to be quite effective for those who maintained the routine. However, the cost of the food substitutes proved a major barrier for most customers who either didn't start or started with good intentions but soon dropped out. John came across as somewhat of a 'timewaster' to Patrick. Nonetheless, Patrick wanted to go through the motions and encourage John to take up the programme or at least to watch the DVD to increase his motivation.

Celestina and the impending pre-diabetes

The scenario: Celestina had experienced a number of episodes of vaginal thrush in the preceding six months. Her pharmacist Sara had insisted she see a doctor about her symptoms, after Celestina had come in asking for yet another tube of clotrimazole cream. In fact, Celestina's doctor Andrew had subsequently found her to be hyperglycaemic when he had checked her blood glucose on the first and a subsequent visit. Celestina felt devastated on hearing this news and could not accept that she was heading towards diabetes. Her brother has had diabetes all of his adult life and Celestina did not want to follow in his footsteps. She returned to the pharmacy a month after her last visit to ask Sara about advice on how to avoid getting 'full-blown diabetes'. She was surprised to find the solution being offered was as simple as a diet and exercise plan.

Presenting complaint: Celestina was recently diagnosed with pre-diabetes or borderline diabetes, as her doctor had called it. She was visiting the pharmacy to speak to Sara. She wanted to find out if there was a way of avoiding diabetes in the long term.

History of presenting complaint: Celestina had been experiencing quite a number of thrush episodes over the summer months, which she had put down to the heat and the 'rushing around, looking after the children'. Her pharmacist had insisted she saw the doctor about the recurring episodes, which together with Celestina's constant tiredness, were beginning to ring some alarm bells. Celestina's glycosylated haemoglobin level (HbA1c) had been found to be 6.4%, which together with other test results, her doctor had interpreted as a sign of borderline diabetes. Celestina was visiting the pharmacist for advice as Sara had spotted the problem in the first place and the doctor hadn't given any specific advice she felt she could follow.

Social context: Celestina was a 45-year-old mother of three. Her children were all under eight years of age. Celestina found it quite challenging coping with the school and nursery runs and other hectic aspects of being a stay-at-home mum. However, she preferred staying at home to the even more chaotic life she had led as a wine-taster before the children were born. Originally from Puerto Rico, she weighed 78 kg and was 167 cm tall, with a BMI of 28, making her 'overweight' for her age. Her husband was of Mediterranean origin and they lived in a semi-detached town house on

Rochester Row, in the fashionable area of the town. Celestina's brother, who was clinically obese, had suffered from diabetes since the age of 21.

Cognitive context: Celestina had not seen a connection between her tiredness and the numerous episodes of thrush that she had experienced over the summer. On her recent visit to the doctor, he had warned her that she would need to start taking tablets to control her blood sugar levels unless she could 'bring things back to normal herself'. This had really scared Celestina. She had to have injections for gestational diabetes (diabetes during pregnancy) some years back, experiencing fluctuations in her blood sugar levels as a result – she was afraid the same would happen if she started taking tablets. In addition, her mother-in-law had recently commented that 'it was downhill all the way once anyone started taking drugs for diabetes'. After speaking to the pharmacist, she thought that perhaps she could join the mums' running club on Thursdays. She hoped her husband would understand as it seemed Celestina also needed to make a number of changes to their evening meals – not forgetting their practice of having wine with dinner each night.

Medication history: No prescribed medication but she had been on insulin for gestational diabetes four years earlier. No known drug allergies. No non-routine vaccinations. She had used several tubes of clotrimazole 2% cream in the past few months. No complementary or alternative medicines.

Dietary information: During the working week, Celestina looked after everyone's meals. The children had cereal before being driven to nursery or school. On her return home, Celestina would have a leisurely breakfast while catching up with news on the 24-hour television channels. This meant she usually skipped lunch, focusing instead on preparing different meals they all enjoyed later in the day. The children would have home-cooked, meat- or poultry-based dishes while Celestina and her husband would eat either traditional Puerto Rican dishes based on legumes and peppers with chorizo sausages or, on occasions, Mediterranean salads with bread. Celestina and her husband ate late, after putting the children to bed and meals in the evening were always accompanied by a glass of Chilean or Mexican Merlot wine.

Pharmacist's perspective: Sara had been qualified for over 10 years. She was not running any specific services aimed at patients with pre-diabetes but knew there was an obligation for her to keep up with advice in relation to diabetes and its prevention. She had attended a postgraduate evening course on the subject in the past year and was keen to exercise her learning. One of the things she wanted to get across to Celestina was that diet and exercise needed to be taken seriously but that this should not put her off trying – Celestina needed to lose around 11% of her weight to restore her BMI to a healthy level and she needed to combine this with frequent and continued exercise. Celestina also needed to start taking greater care of her body, as she now also had a predisposition to a number of other risks normally associated with diabetes. Based on what she had recently learnt, Sara had tried to engage Celestina in a conversation about goal-setting – she wanted to encourage her to choose activities that were specific, doable and, as she called it, forgiving, for example, for her to 'walk for 30 minutes, five days each week'. She also wanted Celestina to benefit from reaching some short-term goals so that she would 'succeed with success'. She thought smaller, consecutive goals would allow Celestina to move ahead in small steps (to eventually reach a distant point) but also that the consecutive feeling of reaching these goals would keep the overall effort invigorated. She therefore wanted to set some two-weekly weight-loss targets. She thought Celestina could give herself small rewards (not food or drink!) on achieving these targets. Celestina was quite happy to keep a self-checking diary. The final part of the conversation between Celestina and Sara revolved around the idea of cue control. Sara wanted Celestina to identify for herself the sorts of environmental or social cues that usually led to undesired eating for her – she could use her diary to identify these and then try to change the association between eating those foods and the particular cue.

Lisa and the longstanding smoking habit

The scenario: Lisa was having a bad winter. A series of lung infections and worsening shortness of breath had led to lung collapse this month. Having now left the hospital she was determined to seek some help to finally give up smoking. On discharge, she had been told to see her general practitioner, who would either refer her to a specialist smoking cessation service or would prescribe the medication Lisa needed to help her quit smoking. However, Lisa recently found out that she was pregnant with her sixth child. On that basis, her GP was reluctant to prescribe any medication for her, asking her instead to try giving up 'drug-free'. Lisa came to the local pharmacy near her estate to find out if the pharmacist had a different view.

Presenting complaint: Lisa's lung had collapsed. She wanted to find out if the pharmacy had anything to help her give up smoking, which she saw as the cause of her illness.

History of presenting complaint: Lisa had experienced excruciating pain earlier this month. Her lung had collapsed and she had spent two weeks in hospital. She had been discharged home with a diagnosis of chronic obstructive pulmonary disease and mild emphysema. She was devastated. Her latest pregnancy meant that her doctor was unwilling to prescribe her any medication to help her give up smoking.

Social context: Lisa was 42 years old and looked after her children fulltime. At one point she had cleaned houses and offices as a part-time, cash-in-hand job. She weighed 63 kg and was 162 cm tall with a BMI of 24, which returned a 'healthy weight'. Lisa was of Irish origin and lived in a small flat on the second floor of a council estate, overlooking the motorway.

Her children were aged 21, 18, 15 and 7 years old. Another child, who would have been five, had suffered cot death when she was three months old. Lisa lived with her two younger children and her dog. None of the children's fathers was in touch with the family. Lisa found her life difficult. Her two eldest daughters had moved out and were living in different flats on the same estate. Both were unemployed and Lisa's eldest daughter had two sons of her own. Lisa had smoked since the age of 12 and had never been able to quit, even while pregnant.

Cognitive context: Lisa felt as though her entire world had fallen apart on hearing that she had chronic obstructive pulmonary disease with mild emphysema. Although she had an existing diagnosis of asthma, she had viewed this as a mild condition, not thinking for a moment that it would lead to anything more sinister. She was completely devastated. She had seen people with chronic lung conditions around her estate, confined to their balconies, oxygen always by their side. She had thought that the chest infections, constant phlegm and wheezing had been a result of the harsh winter. She simply had to try and give up smoking but it would be difficult because she had allowed her 15-year-old son to start smoking in the house. Now, to make matters worse, she had found out that she was pregnant for the sixth time. This meant that the doctor would not prescribe anything to help her on her way. Lisa felt both scared and angry. She thought that perhaps the pharmacist, who usually supplied her with her inhalers, would be able to 'prescribe' a product to help her.

Medication history: Before her admission to hospital, Lisa had been using salbutamol inhaler as required, mometasone dry powder inhaler 200 µg twice daily, and salmeterol dry powder for inhalation 50 µg 2 puffs twice daily, for asthma. Since her discharge from hospital, ipratropium 20 µg inhaler, 2 puffs four times daily had been added to her list of medicines. No known drug allergies. She had received an influenza vaccine and a pneumococcal vaccine while in the hospital. No current non-prescription medication. No complementary or alternative medicines.

Dietary information: Lisa ate a diet of carbohydrate and meats. She found it hard to feed the family more than three cooked meals a week and often resorted to using snacks and sandwiches to get by. Her appetite in the last month had vastly diminished, which she now realised might have been a result of the pregnancy as well as her illness.

Pharmacist's perspective: Lisa was well known to Tony, the pharmacist, who had worked at that particular branch of the company for over four years. Tony had qualified for providing specialist one-to-one support for smoking cessation by completing a formal training course. He now dedicated two hours a day to seeing patients as part of an NHS Stop Smoking support service, commissioned by the local primary care trust. His clients were normally either referred via their GP or walked through the door after seeing the service advertised on the shop window. His service was based on behavioural support and Tony made sure he conducted all the initial consultations himself, taking a full history from all clients so that he could devise a bespoke programme to meet individuals' needs. With a range of medication available for Tony to supply, he felt the service was really meeting the needs of the community in this deprived part of the city. Patients were normally asked to return every week for a month and then every fortnight. Those who managed to give up smoking mostly did so within 12 weeks of starting the programme. Lisa's case was different. Tony had been told that nicotine replacement products should only be used in pregnancy as an absolute last resort. He thought perhaps she could go 'cold turkey' and proceeded to provide her with general advice:

- Set a quit date.
- Tell her family and friends that she planned to quit.
- Anticipate and plan for the challenges she would face while quitting.
- Remove cigarettes and other tobacco products from her home and other environments.
- Come back and tell the pharmacist about her progress.

Tony also thought that Lisa could try managing her cravings by reducing the association with other activities such as eating, drinking alcohol and smoking with friends or family members.

Kenneth and Alistair and the hidden alcohol habit

The scenario: Kenneth's son, Alistair, had been in a state of constant worry for the past three months. His father was being discharged from hospital. On the way home, they stopped by the local pharmacy because Alistair wanted to buy his father a hot-water bottle. Kenneth was feeling achy and weary and Alistair wanted something to help give his ill father some comfort. The pharmacy was offering an alcohol screening service according to the posters displayed outside and near the counter. Alistair found it a cruel irony to see this information now that his father had already suffered the full effects of an apparent hidden alcohol problem. Tony, the pharmacist, noticed Alistair's interest in his new service and asked if he wanted to complete a short quiz to find out what the service was about. Alistair thought for a moment and asked if he could take the quiz away with him instead. His father lived around the corner and it would be he who would have most benefited from such a service. Once inside, Alistair was mortified by his own answers to the questions in the quiz.

Presenting complaint: Kenneth had been admitted to hospital for the second time in three months, with late-stage cirrhosis of the liver as a result of a longstanding addiction to alcohol, something that none of his family had seemed to recognise beforehand.

History of presenting complaint: When Kenneth's son had seen him three months earlier, Kenneth looked as though he had developed a 'beer belly' but his face had been haggard and gaunt. Soon after, he had been admitted to hospital and diagnosed as having cirrhosis of the liver – the 'beer belly' had been a result of fluid around his abdomen because of damage to his liver. He had been sent home but had then had further problems with his bowels, urine and some confusion. He had been admitted to hospital for the second time and was now returning home.

Social context: Kenneth was 66 years old. He had been a labourer for 37 years before giving up work upon his wife's death four years previously. He weighed 85 kg and was 179 cm tall, which made him 'overweight' with a BMI of 26.5 – but in fact, most of the extra weight had amassed around Kenneth's abdomen and was related to the fluid of the ascites. His appearance otherwise was that of an emaciated, old man. Kenneth was of Scottish origin. He lived on his own but now his son was arranging for his sister (Alistair's aunt) to come and stay and look after him. Kenneth's job had been hard but it had kept him busy. Since his wife's death, Kenneth had tried to keep himself occupied but to relieve the loneliness in the evening he normally had a glass or two of Scottish ale. His son Alistair was 34 and worked for an advertising company and lived in a town 50 miles away.

Cognitive context: Kenneth had been suffering from a number of ailments of late and just wanted it all to be over, 'one way or another'. As far as he was concerned, life without his wife had been almost unbearable in itself and now the discomfort created by his expanding list of conditions made it impossible for him to cope. To make matters worse he had heard the doctors talk about him having an addiction to alcohol – had they even put him on tablets to stop him from having any more ale? The final humiliation was being taken home by his son and being told that his sister would be staying to look after him. Alistair was worried about his father. Having in effect left Kenneth to look after himself alone for the past few years, he was trying to do his best to help him now. The alcohol screening service offered by the pharmacy had caught Alistair's eye. When he looked at what the pharmacist had called a 'quiz', it proved a real eye-opener about his own relationship with alcohol. Work meant having to take clients out two to three times a week, when he would consume more than five or six drinks per night – and, yes, of course, at times he had a feeling of guilt after drinking and, yes, he was from time to time unable to remember the exact details of the evening before. Did this mean that he too had an alcohol addiction?

Medication history: Kenneth was sent home on amiloride and hydro-chlorothiazide tablets (2.5 mg/ 25 mg) two daily, ascorbic acid 500 mg tablets two daily, thiamine 50 mg tablets two daily, vitamin B tablets compound strong (nicotinamide 20 mg, pyridoxine hydrochloride 2 mg, riboflavin 2 mg, thiamine hydrochloride 5 mg) one tablet three times a day, simvastatin 10 mg tablets one at night, propranolol 80 mg tablets twice a day, lactulose 30 mL three times a day, and disulfiram 200 mg tablets one daily. No known drug allergies. No non-routine vaccinations. No current non-prescription medication. No complementary or alternative medicines.

Dietary information: Kenneth normally had oats or porridge in the morning, some bread and cheese or cold meats for lunch and, for dinner, either eggs or tinned soup at home or fried fish and chips when he wanted a bought, cooked meal. His appetite had drastically reduced in the past five months so that he was only eating about a third of his usual food intake. Shopping was as required from a low-cost local supermarket and the local off-licence. Kenneth had been having a glass or two of Scottish ale every night.

Pharmacist's perspective: Stewart had recently signed up to deliver an alcohol screening and brief intervention service in his pharmacy, with the backing of the local healthcare cooperative. He was keen for customers to complete a questionnaire called 'AUDIT' which enabled him to assess if they were hazardous, harmful or dependent drinkers. Stewart would then either offer general education or a brief intervention and even follow-up monitoring depending on patients' level of risk – he was also able to make referrals to a local harm-reduction team if needed. The intervention was based around providing information on the benefits of reducing alcohol consumption (e.g., improved memory, better sleep, less risk of cancer and liver damage), goals to aim for (i.e., safe drinking limits depending on the customer) and strategies for reducing alcohol consumption (e.g., changing social habits, having smaller drinks, exploring new interests). Stewart was particularly impressed with the small, laminated card that patients could be given to take away, which presented some general advice in an easy-to-digest format. But the uptake of the service had been slow. It wasn't the incentive of payments for the service so much as his personal conviction that it would genuinely help people that was driving Stewart to push the service at every opportunity. He'd realised recently that using the 'short readiness to change questionnaire' (SRTCQ) was potentially a better route to getting people interested and was trying to refine the way he could opportunistically ask people questions such as whether the amount they drank had changed over the past three months, whether they were interested in drinking less and whether they thought they normally drink more than they should. He had experienced modest success over the past week using this technique but normally resorted to offering the questionnaire to customers for self-completion instead.

Dinesh and the risk of heart disease

The scenario: Dinesh had been sent out by his wife to buy a pack of nappies from the pharmacy chain in the local parade of shops. He felt sleepy and exhausted – the arrival of their first baby was taking its toll on him. The pharmacy was offering a healthy heart service. Dinesh would never normally consider taking part in such a service, but somehow the thought of rushing back to the flat did not fill him with excitement either. One of the questions that the leaflet describing the service asked was, 'Have you been feeling tired and lethargic?' Dinesh certainly had felt worn-out for the past few months – the leaflet made him think. He didn't need much persuasion when the counter assistant asked Dinesh if he wanted to take up the offer of the healthy heart service. The pharmacist, Sheila, smiled at Dinesh and pointed the way to the consultation room. There was a consent form to complete and then some questions about Dinesh, before she could proceed to take the measurements from him. Half an hour later and clutching his test results, Dinesh felt devastated and in more despair – he had just been told he was at risk of coronary heart disease.

Presenting complaint: Dinesh had been feeling tired for months. On a visit to the pharmacy, he had taken the spontaneous decision to take part in the healthy heart service being offered on the premises.

History of presenting complaint: Dinesh was exhausted. As well as the sleepless nights, looking after his wife and their new baby, Dinesh knew he had been neglecting his diet and failing to take adequate exercise. A few months earlier, he had lost his permanent post at the local police station and had been left instead with short stints of menial administration work. With the birth of the baby imminent, Dinesh had found it difficult to cope with the reduced salary and the loss of status. He had taken to eating junk food and watching television in the evenings as a way of coping with what he saw as the demise of his career and the loss of his identity.

Social context: Dinesh was 45 years old and worked as a relief administrator at the local police station. He weighed 74 kg and was 172 cm tall, which made him just 'overweight' with a BMI of 25.01. Dinesh was of mixed Anglo-Indian origin and lived with his wife and new baby in a small flat in south London. He had worked in the local police station as a constable for six years before taking voluntary redundancy. Dinesh's baby was three weeks old.

Cognitive context: After a series of disappointing appraisals, Dinesh had been placed under pressure to take voluntary redundancy from his post as a police constable. However, as they had been short-staffed in other areas at the station, Dinesh had been offered relief work as an administrator. Reduced to doing paperwork his colleagues did not want to complete, the new line of work left Dinesh feeling inadequate and even emasculated. He had resorted to comfort food in the evenings as a way of coping. The arrival of the baby and the sleepless nights had only made matters worse. Feeling exhausted and worn-out, something about the healthy heart service appealed to him. The pharmacist had measured Dinesh's blood pressure, waist circumference, height and weight, blood cholesterol and blood glucose, and Dinesh had enjoyed the attention he had received during the consultation. However, afterwards the pharmacist had told him that in the next 10 years his 'risk of coronary heart disease' was at best 1 in 10 and at worst 1 in 5. She had provided some other basic information relating to diet and exercise but had not described anything Dinesh didn't already know. His father had recently undergone a double-bypass despite years of dieting and exercise – Dinesh felt doomed. He rubbed the palm of his hands on his eyes and face, took a minute to compose himself then thanked the pharmacist and left, clutching the nappies as he made his way home.

Medication history: No prescribed medication. No known drug allergies. No non-routine vaccinations. No current non-prescription medication. No complementary or alternative medicines.

Dietary information: Before the baby was born, Dinesh's diet had become a quick breakfast of coffee and toast most mornings, lunch was often sandwiches at work and dinner a meal of pasta or pizza followed by crisps and chocolates while watching television with his wife. Since the birth of his new baby, Dinesh was having meals erratically, keeping hunger away with unhealthy snacks instead.

Pharmacist's perspective: Sheila had been accredited to run the healthy heart service, which screened for the risk of coronary heart disease. The service involved a 20-minute consultation in the pharmacy to measure blood pressure, waist circumference, height and weight, blood cholesterol and blood glucose. Afterwards, she was able not only to return people's raw measurements to them but also to provide them with a prediction of their risk of heart disease as either low, moderate or high. The idea was that she would provide lifestyle information for those at either moderate or high risk of coronary heart disease, in an attempt to help avert the risk.

Cases involving prescribed medication

Mrs Janet Wentworth and tamoxifen

The scenario: Mrs Janet Wentworth was collecting her first prescription for tamoxifen tablets, following the completion of a course of radiotherapy at the local hospital. The wait at the outpatient pharmacy had been over 30 minutes long but Mrs Janet Wentworth didn't mind as she thought it might be a good opportunity to ask some further questions about the tablets she had been prescribed. A technician called out Mrs Janet Wentworth's name, and on sitting down to collect her medicine, she asked politely if instead she could have a 'quick word' with the pharmacist. Jon, a pharmacist, was walking through the busy dispensary and was called to help. He stared at the technician for a moment without speaking, before taking his place to face Mrs Janet Wentworth. In fact, it seemed Mrs Janet Wentworth had a number of questions for Jon, some of which he was unable to answer on the spot. She had been prescribed tamoxifen, which was not a medicine Jon was particularly familiar with. As the conversation continued, Jon sank lower and lower in his seat. Towards the end of the conversation, Jon wondered whether Mrs Janet Wentworth had really wished for a 'quick word' after all.

Presenting complaint: Mrs Janet Wentworth had been prescribed tamoxifen following the removal of a breast lump. On visiting the outpatient pharmacy, she brought up a number of questions for the pharmacist, some of which he was not equipped to answer straightaway.

History of presenting complaint: Mrs Janet Wentworth had been diagnosed with oestrogen-receptor-positive breast cancer six months earlier. She had had surgery to remove the lump and some of the surrounding normal tissue followed by several weeks of radiotherapy. She had been prescribed long-term tamoxifen afterwards and was collecting her first prescription.

Social context: Mrs Janet Wentworth was 45 years old. She had lived with her husband of 22 years until a few months earlier. Mr Wentworth had found the strain of Mrs Wentworth's illness 'too much to cope with' and had moved permanently into his London pied-à-terre, Mrs Wentworth suspected, with his secretary. Mrs Wentworth was now the sole occupant of their five-bedroomed suburban house as both of her children were attending campus-based universities. She weighed 65 kg and was 171 cm tall, with a BMI of 22.2, which made her a 'healthy weight' for her age. Before her illness, she had been working part-time at the local estate agents. She had been granted unpaid leave for nine months and was keen to get back to her post.

Cognitive context: Mrs Wentworth had been severely distressed by her diagnosis but was now determined to 'get her life back' and to re-establish some routine. She had thought that perhaps the pharmacist could be a source of further information about her new tablets, which she had already read about on the internet. At the outpatient pharmacy counter, she had thought it a brilliant opportunity to raise her concerns with a professional rather than consulting the internet or friends as she often did. Mrs Wentworth had to decide whether to go in for a cosmetic procedure to reconstruct some of her breast tissue but had read that tamoxifen could increase the risk of blood clots with surgery and sought reassurance. In fact, Mrs Wentworth believed 'knowing her luck', she was more likely to end up with both blood clots and an unsuccessful operation than any other outcome. Jon and she had also spoken about how to take her medicine. Mrs Wentworth mentioned a friend had recommended taking tamoxifen only every other day because otherwise it would induce hot flushes and bring on early menopause. When Jon had probed further, Mrs Wentworth said that her friend (who was 'only 37 when put on tamoxifen') had remained menopausal even after stopping the course of treatment. Mrs Wentworth told Jon that the 'every other day' dosing really helped her friend, who some days experienced particularly bad hot flushes and sweating, which on other days settled down and all this correlated with the alternate-day dosing.

Medication history: At the time she was prescribed tamoxifen 20 mg tablets, once daily. No known drug allergies. No non-routine vaccinations. No non-prescription medication. She had bought a supplement containing 'soya isoflavones 400 mg' on a friend's recommendation but was unsure whether to take it or not.

Dietary information: Mrs Wentworth believed she had a healthy diet. She shopped at an exclusive supermarket and made sure she had at least five portions of fruit and vegetables each day. In addition, she had home-made fruit 'smoothies' every morning with her breakfast of organic muesli. She did not normally drink alcohol and had only the occasional glass of wine over lunch if she went to the health club.

Pharmacist's perspective: At the time, Jon had been qualified for five years, having conducted his pre-registration year in the same hospital pharmacy. Jon could not remember whether or not tamoxifen really did increase the risk of blood clots but tried to appease Mrs Wentworth's concerns. He thought it would be better to move on to discuss her adherence to what Jon considered to be a straightforward once-daily dose. Although Jon had previously come across unusual patient beliefs in relation to medicine taking, he was really unsure how to tackle Mrs Wentworth's beliefs about the alternate dosing recommended by her friend. In addition, he didn't know the answer to Mrs Wentworth's query regarding the soya isoflavone supplements – but suspected these should not be taken in someone taking anti-oestrogen medication.

Jamilla and her asthma

The scenario: Jamilla had been admitted to St Annabel's hospital via the accident and emergency unit and was now resting on the respiratory (Jasmine) ward. Karen, the pharmacy pre-registration trainee was sent up to Jasmine to take a medication history from Jamilla. Although Jamilla's condition was now stable, she had had severe coughing and shortness of breath, which had necessitated a 999 ambulance call two days earlier. On speaking with Jamilla, Karen soon suspected non-adherence as the main reason for Jamilla's admission. It seemed Jamilla had been strongly influenced by her mother's advice and that of an alternative practitioner regarding the management of her longstanding asthma. Karen wondered if the severe asthma attack would now act as a wake-up call to Jamilla to manage her medication better. Karen made ample notes for her training portfolio and decided to return with the most effective advice after speaking with her pre-registration tutor.

Presenting complaint: Jamilla had had a severe asthma attack while running for the bus two mornings earlier. She had tried using her salbutamol inhaler, to no avail. Luckily, Jamilla's friends were with her and able to call an ambulance immediately.

History of presenting complaint: Jamilla's asthma had been worsening for the past five months. Her mother had recommended a spiritual healer, whom Jamilla had visited for a 'cure'. The healer had recommended a withdrawal of Jamilla's medication, which had finally culminated in a severe asthma attack when Jamilla had attempted to run for the bus two days earlier, on Saturday morning.

Social context: Jamilla was 20 years old and studying for a journalism degree at university. She weighed 69 kg and was 163 cm tall, which made her 'overweight' with a BMI of 26. Jamilla was of Pakistani origin and had been living in a shared student house with five others for the past six months, to save money. She was in the first year of her degree, having taken a year out to retake her A-Levels and to work to build a cash reserve for university. She still worked part-time and some weekends at a fast-food restaurant. Her first-year examinations were imminent and she had been revising hard.

Cognitive context: Jamilla was studying hard for her degree. Her asthma had been worsening in the past five months. Her mother, who had seen Jamilla develop asthma in primary school, had thought it time to try something new. A friend of a friend had visited a spiritual healer for a similar condition, so Jamilla's mum had obtained the contact details and suggested strongly that Jamilla also visited for a 'cure'. The healer had promised Jamilla that she could channel healing energies by passing her hands over Jamilla's body, saying that her other asthmatic patients had all derived benefits from spiritual healing of that nature. Some of Jamilla's friends from home were medical students and Jamilla had decided to speak to them about her experience, not to seek their advice but to broaden their horizons. Jamilla's friends were horrified to hear about the approach she had taken. To her friends, asthma was closely related to dust mites, which produced a very powerful allergen that worsened asthma. Yet, Jamilla had continued to visit the spiritual healer and taken her advice to come off her inhalers as a trial. Although she still carried her salbutamol inhaler with her, she had begun to feel better after a few sessions and, before her admission, had been starting to think that her asthma was 'now a thing of the past'.

Medication history: Prior to her admission, Jamilla had been prescribed salbutamol 100 µg as required and budesonide 400 µg twice daily. After emergency management of her severe acute asthma, Jamilla was now on a reducing dose of prednisolone, her corticosteroid inhaler had been changed to fluticasone propionate 500 µg twice daily and salmeterol 100 µg twice daily had been added to her regimen. No known drug allergies. No non-routine vaccinations. No current non-prescription medication. No complementary or alternative medicines but she had been to see an alternative practitioner for the past month.

Dietary information: Jamilla lived on a diet of cereal, pasta, noodles, cheese and takeaways. Lunch was normally from the student union shop with dinner made at home, on a shared rota with her housemates. When working, Jamilla had her meals at work. Jamilla's family home was 20 miles away and she sometimes visited for traditional meals cooked by her mother or older sisters.

Pharmacist's perspective: Karen was a diligent, hard-working pre-registration student, who was keen to put both the practice and the science of pharmacy into use during her training. She tried hard not to make any judgements about Jamilla personally but couldn't help feeling a certain degree of incomprehension at Jamilla's careless approach to her medication management. Although traumatic, Karen hoped Jamilla had learnt a good lesson now and would never try experimenting with her medicines again. She also wanted to provide Jamilla with some further effective advice but was unsure how to package the information in a way that would convince Jamilla about the benefits of sticking to the medical approach. Karen thought that perhaps consulting her pre-registration tutor would be a good start.

Henry and his tablets

The scenario: In February 2012, Mr Henry Evans was referred to the practice pharmacy for a Medicines Use Review (MUR) by the general practitioner, Dr Timmins. Dr Timmins had recently employed a practice pharmacist, Mrs Toulson, and was keen to ensure all eligible patients received an MUR where warranted. It was normally Mrs Tracey Evans (Henry Evans's wife) who booked in to see Dr Timmins. She was an elderly, frail lady, who had had Alzheimer's disease for the past few years, and Henry would bring her in every now and then, either for a check-up or to talk through her deteriorating condition. On this occasion, Mr Evans had also mentioned his own health, albeit in passing. Mrs Toulson booked an appointment for Mr Evans and was at first surprised to find both Mr and Mrs Evans arriving for the MUR. Nonetheless, she began the consultation by asking Mr Evans to go through his daily routine, providing as much information as he wanted. Mr Evans explained that he would need to be quick as it was difficult to keep his wife sitting still for longer than 10 minutes.

Presenting complaint: Mr Evans had chronic heart failure. On a recent visit to his GP, he mentioned that he had been having trouble helping his wife Tracey in the house, the work was physically exhausting and he often felt out of breath and unable to cope.

History of presenting complaint: Mr Evans had been diagnosed with chronic heart failure seven years earlier. He had been stabilised on a range of medication but when he mentioned a recent decline in his condition, instead of changing his regimen, his GP had wondered whether Mr Evans had been taking his medication as prescribed. Dr Timmins had referred his patient to the practice pharmacist for an MUR.

Social context: Mr Evans was 85 years old and lived at home with his wife of 60 years in a small cottage in the centre of town. He weighed 64 kg and was 186 cm tall, which made him borderline 'underweight' with a BMI of 18.5. Mr Evans was of English origin. Before retiring, he had worked as a government tax inspector. He had spent the past seven years looking after his wife, who had developed Alzheimer's disease and now could not be left 'alone even for five minutes in one day'. Apart from reluctantly accepting mobile meals, Mr Evans refused other help offered by the local social services, preferring to look after his wife himself in their home.

Cognitive context: Mr Evans thought he was quite competent to look after both himself and his wife. He had first been diagnosed with chronic heart failure when he was 78, which had come 'as a real blow' to him because, after years of service, he had been looking forward to a healthy and happy retirement with his wife. Her disease had now progressed to such an extent that it almost necessitated 24-hour supervision. Nonetheless, Mr Evans persevered, as he didn't dare think of the option of placing Mrs Evans in a care home. Mr Evans had been prescribed a number of medicines, most of which were to be taken in the morning. However, one tablet had been prescribed as a twice-daily dose and Mr Evans often 'forgot' to take the latter dose if he was busy with looking after Tracey in the evenings. As far as he was concerned, this had not 'done him any harm'. He put his breathlessness and recent discomfort down to his wife's deteriorating condition.

Medication history: At the time, Mr Evans had been prescribed enalapril 10 mg twice daily, aspirin 75 mg every morning and bendroflumethiazide 5 mg every morning. No known drug allergies. No non-routine vaccinations. No current non-prescription medication. No complementary or alternative medicines.

Dietary information: Mr Evans still managed to conduct some of the shopping by visiting his local grocery shop, although he did resort to using a local council mobile meals service three times a week. When he cooked, the meals were normally quickly prepared, humble soups or meat dishes. His wife's appetite had decreased considerably over the past few months and he was cooking smaller portions to reduce unnecessary wastage.

Pharmacist's perspective: Mrs Toulson had received the MUR referral from Dr Timmins. It appeared that on speaking with Mr Evans, Dr Timmins had uncovered potential medication adherence issues. As Mr Evans was on a diuretic, considered a high-risk medication, Mrs Toulson saw this as an excellent opportunity to prove her expertise as the practice pharmacist. As the conversation unfolded, Mrs Toulson began to appreciate Mr Evans's position. Two minutes in, Mrs Evans began asking him a series of seemingly redundant and unconnected questions, which took away his attention and made a coherent conversation with Mrs Toulson near impossible. Nonetheless, Mrs Toulson managed to unearth the patient's medication beliefs and thought up an easy plan to resolve his adherence issues. However, she needed to speak with Dr Timmins first as the solution required a change to Mr Evans's prescription.

Bethany and the 'steroid' cream

The scenario: Mrs Hirst seemed hesitant to collect her daughter's prescription for hydrocortisone cream and asked if she could have a chat with the pharmacist. She had visited the local pharmacy several times in the past month, asking advice about emollient creams and baby bathing products as recommended by her GP. Now, she was visiting the outpatient dispensary of her local hospital following a visit to a consultant dermatologist. Mrs Hirst's daughter Bethany had developed eczema, which was not improving and was now severely disrupting her night-time sleep. Mrs Hirst's GP had refused to prescribe a corticosteroid cream, saying that the disadvantages, such as the thinning of the skin, outweighed any advantage a corticosteroid cream could bring. She had asked Mrs Hirst to persevere with the emollient regimen. However, a consultant dermatologist who had seen Bethany that morning had convinced Mrs Hirst to try a short course of hydrocortisone cream. According to the consultant, if used correctly, there was very little risk from corticosteroid applied as a cream. Mrs Hirst was confused and riddled with guilt and just wanted to do the best for her baby.

Presenting complaint: Bethany, an otherwise healthy and thriving baby, had had eczema for the past month. Her mother had come to the outpatient pharmacy to collect a prescription for hydrocortisone cream after visiting a consultant dermatologist.

History of presenting complaint: Bethany had not been sleeping well at night because of eczema that affected patchy areas on her chest and head, including a small area on her face. Her mother had been smothering her in an emollient cream prescribed by the GP and also attempting to put mittens on her to prevent scratching at night. She was also using an oil-based product in Bethany's baths and aqueous cream instead of soap. Yet Bethany's eczema had worsened and this had meant a return to broken night-time sleep for Bethany as well as Mr and Mrs Hirst.

Social context: Bethany was delivered at full term, weighing 3.4 kg (7.5 lb), placing her on the 50th centile on the new UK–WHO growth chart for girls. At five months, she weighed 7.5 kg (16.5 lb), which was on the 75th centile and this meant that she had developed well in the past few months. Her mother, Mrs Hirst, was on maternity leave from her job as a primary school teacher and her father continued to work as an accountant. Both Mr and Mrs Hirst were of English origin, although Mrs Hirst's ancestors were French. The couple and their then small kitten had moved into a new-build, three-bedroomed house 18 months before Bethany had been born. Mrs Hirst had made quite a number of friends through antenatal classes, which provided great peer support and parenting advice.

Cognitive context: Mrs Hirst wanted to be the perfect mum and until Bethany's eczema had felt happy and in control. She had breast-fed Bethany fulltime for three months. Then she had started weaning Bethany on baby rice, slowly adding what she considered to be 'non-allergenic' foods, a little at a time. At four months, Bethany had been established on a range of these simple foods. Then Mrs Hirst had noticed a small rash on her daughter's stomach, which had quickly grown to several small patches on her chest and head, and even a small area on her face. Horrified that she had introduced the 'wrong food', Mrs Hirst had quickly taken her daughter back to just having breast milk and baby rice but to no avail. Her friends had advised changing the washing power to one without colour, fragrance or biological enzymes, which again had not had any impact on Bethany's eczema. After trialling a series of creams recommended by her antenatal friends, Mrs Hirst had taken Bethany to the doctor for advice. The doctor had encouraged Mrs Hirst to continue with one particular emollient, in addition prescribing a bath oil and aqueous cream, instead of soap or shampoo for Bethany's bath times. The doctor had confirmed Mrs Hirst's fear that a corticosteroid cream at this age would have far too many disadvantages to make it worth a try. But instead of improving, in fact Bethany's eczema was getting slightly worse. One of Mrs Hirst's friends admitted she had resorted to using a corticosteroid cream on her older child some years back, on the recommendation of a consultant dermatologist, and that it had worked a miracle, permanently curing the eczema after a few days. Using her husband's private health insurance, Mrs Hirst had booked an appointment with a consultant dermatologist. The consultant was indeed recommending a short course of hydrocortisone cream to Mrs Hirst, saying its advantages would outweigh the disadvantages if used correctly.

Medication history: At the time, Mrs Hirst had been recommended to use an emollient cream on Bethany's skin, an oil-based product for her baths and aqueous cream instead of soap by the GP. The new prescription for Bethany was for hydrocortisone cream, 1%, to be applied thinly over the affected areas twice daily. No known drug allergies. No non-routine vaccinations. No current non-prescription medication. No complementary or alternative medicines.

Dietary information: Bethany had been breast-fed fully and had yet to consume any powdered formula milk. Her mother had started weaning her on baby rice at three months followed by apples, bananas, pears, sweet potatoes, carrots and peas. Mrs Hirst was yet to introduce meat or dairy products to Bethany's diet. Since Bethany's eczema had erupted, she was on breast milk and baby rice only.

Pharmacist's perspective: Mrs Chong was an experienced dispensary pharmacist, and herself a mother to four young children. When Mrs Hirst asked to speak with her about the hydrocortisone cream newly prescribed for her daughter, Mrs Chong felt a great degree of empathy. She too had been left with the same quandary when her fourth child had unexpectedly developed eczema as a small baby. In fact, Mrs Chong, who kept her continuing professional development records diligently up-to-date, had recently attended a postgraduate training course on skin conditions, and had a chart to hand in the dispensary, which helped explain the correct amount of corticosteroid to apply to eczematous skin. Mrs Chong nodded to Mrs Hirst and sat down to explain the 'finger-tip-unit' using the chart as a basis for the discussions. Mrs Hirst was to estimate the area of eczema and use the equivalent of one 'finger-tip-unit' (amount of cream expelled from the tube to cover from the tip of her index finger to the first crease) to cover an area twice the size of her hand. Mrs Hirst looked surprised and puzzled all at the same time. Mrs Chong wanted to explain that using this measure, instead of just applying the corticosteroid cream thinly as the doctor would have advised, had been proven to reduce the risk of side-effects.

Sylvia and her new anticoagulant treatment

The scenario: Sylvia was referred to the pharmacist by the counter assistant, as a potential candidate for a consultation under the New Medicines Service (NMS) arrangements. Sylvia had just been discharged from hospital with warfarin tablets following a pulmonary embolism. Although she had an appointment to go back to the hospital in a week's time, she had become confused about which tablets to take from three packs provided to her on discharge from the hospital. The pharmacist, Mary, was only too happy to recruit Sylvia to the service. She asked for her consent and then proceeded to ask Sylvia some pre-set questions to initiate the conversation. To her surprise, she found Sylvia had forgotten which of the warfarin tablets she was to take for the next week. What's more, she had misplaced her yellow warfarin card and, although appreciative of the seriousness of her condition, Sylvia seemed to have very little knowledge about lifestyle factors, and drug and food interactions to avoid while on warfarin. After the consultation, which had necessitated a phone-call to the hospital, Mary arranged to see Sylvia again in three weeks' time to check on her progress.

Presenting complaint: Sylvia had been discharged from hospital with three different packs of warfarin tablets, none of which had any instructions written on them. She could not remember which one she had been told to take until next week.

History of presenting complaint: About two weeks earlier, Sylvia had woken in the night with excruciating pain in her chest on the right-hand side.

Her husband Antony had driven her to hospital, fearing the worst. After a few hours, the doctors had discovered a large pulmonary embolism in Sylvia's right lung, for which they had initiated therapy with low molecular weight heparin. After a two-week stay on the ward, Sylvia had been discharged on warfarin and told to return to the anticoagulant clinic the following week.

Social context: Sylvia was 55 years old and had taken early retirement following surgical treatment for uterine prolapse eight weeks earlier. She weighed 89 kg and was 170 cm tall, which made her 'obese' with a BMI of 30.8. Sylvia was of Italian origin and lived with her husband in a modest terraced house. She had worked as a doctor's receptionist before her retirement. Her husband was still working – he was an electrician for a local 24-hour electrical emergency firm. Their five children had all left home and there were five grandchildren living nearby.

Cognitive context: Having worked at the doctor's surgery, Sylvia considered herself quite 'medication savvy'. Although she had kept an old copy of the *British National Formulary* from her job at the surgery, on getting home she could not work out what she was meant to be taking the next day, no matter how many times she tried to read the section on warfarin. Over the years, she had appreciated the work of the local pharmacists and when she encountered problems with her own prescription after leaving hospital this time, the pharmacy was her first port of call. Sylvia had been diagnosed with a prolapsed uterus the previous year after suffering from stress incontinence, lower backache, and problems with her bowel movements. This had upset Sylvia a great deal at the time and eventually she had undergone reconstructive surgery six weeks prior to the pulmonary embolism. She was horrified to think that she could have died as a result of the embolism but at least grateful that it had been discovered and treated in time. She had vowed to do everything in her power to get her health back to normal again. She certainly didn't want to ruin her chances of a 'proper recovery' by not taking her warfarin tablets correctly. But, no matter how hard she tried, all she could remember was being given a bag with 1-mg, 3-mg and 5-mg warfarin tablets and an appointment card for a consultation with the anticoagulant clinic in a week's time. She had been given a yellow card and told to read it for medication and foods to avoid, but she had since misplaced the card and could not find it anywhere.

Medication history: Sylvia had been given a range of warfarin tablets and told to take one 3-mg warfarin tablet at the same time each day, although she could not remember this information, given to her earlier in the day. No known drug allergies. No non-routine vaccinations. No current non-prescription medication. No complementary or alternative medicines.

Dietary information: Sylvia had a rich diet of pasta and breads and took pride in her Italian cooking, which often saw her and her husband eating late dinners accompanied by chianti and followed by dessert. When the grandchildren came to stay, Sylvia often finished their leftovers as she did not like to see food go to waste. She had been warned about her weight over the years and was thinking of making changes to her diet after discharge from the hospital.

Pharmacist's perspective: Mary was a relatively young pharmacist. She took a great deal of responsibility for her own learning and was keen to be the best possible pharmacist in her new job. She still recalled some very important facts about warfarin from her university studies and had recently undertaken training to provide the NMS. It seemed inconceivable to her that Sylvia had been discharged from hospital without clear guidance on how to take her warfarin, and most importantly what food and medicine to avoid. Going through her list of questions for the NMS, Mary was able to establish that Sylvia was in fact very much intending to adhere to her medication but she genuinely did not remember the dose. In addition, Mary also discovered Sylvia's intention to start making drastic changes to her diet, which was not recommended on newly starting a medicine such as warfarin. She asked Sylvia if she would mind sharing the detail of her medical team and ward at the hospital so that she could make enquiries about her warfarin dose as a first step to helping her. She thought it would also be vital to meet with Sylvia again in three weeks' time to make sure that she was not experiencing any further issues with her warfarin after visiting the anticoagulant clinic.

8

Research case studies

Teaching notes

Educational objectives

This second case study chapter is designed to support the reader's learning of social and cognitive pharmacy research and its interrelationship with existing psychosocial knowledge. Nowadays, all those who practise pharmacy in whatever setting will in some way come into contact with research, whether it is through having to read and interpret others' research or indeed having to conduct research as a component of their own work. This final chapter aims to help the reader recognise the application of the two approaches to knowledge construction (epistemologies) discussed in Chapter 2. It also aims to provide the reader with an opportunity to identify the methods that have been applied to generate research outlined in the hypothetical cases. The ultimate aim is to help readers develop their understanding of the relationship between a particular epistemology and a particular research method, type of data and accompanying analyses. One consistent criticism of pharmacy practice research is its tentative links with existing psychosocial theory, be it theory as impetus for the research or in explaining what bearing the research findings have on existing theory. Therefore, another aim of the current chapter is to help readers identify any interrelationship the case may have with existing knowledge. The chapter is aimed mainly towards those at Level 3/4 onwards, where readers might be contemplating their own pharmacy research.

Learning outcomes

The following learning outcomes are anticipated as a result of successfully completing the tasks in relation to the cases outlined in this chapter:

- Level 3 readers will be able to *criticise* the relationship between the research and existing psychosocial theory.

- Level 3 readers will be able to *analyse* the relationship between the approach to knowledge construction, the research methods used and the data generated.
- Level 4 readers will be able to *compare and contrast* opposing epistemologies applied to the investigation.
- Level 4 readers will be able to *question* the epistemological approach taken by the researchers.

Tasks

The following tasks accompany each case presented in this chapter. All readers are recommended to work through all of the tasks to fully benefit from the learning objectives.

Level 3: criticise the relationship between the research and existing psychosocial theory

Use the following questions to help you establish some of the basic facts in each case. Then refer to the case scenario and, where necessary, use quotations or paraphrase to form and express a judgement about your conclusion.

- Has existing and established theory been used as impetus for the research?
- Have the research findings been explicitly interrelated to existing theory in the field?

Level 3: analyse the relationship between the approach to knowledge construction, the research methods used and the data generated

Use the following questions to help you establish some of the basic facts in each case. Then refer to the case scenario and where necessary use quotations or paraphrase to present a valid argument to support your conclusion.

- What is the epistemological approach implied by the research detailed in the case?
- What are the research methods that have been used in the case?
- What is the type of data that has been generated by the research?
- Are the approaches to knowledge construction, research methods and data congruent?

Level 4: compare and contrast opposing epistemologies applied to the investigation

Use the following questions to help you identify the opposing epistemological approach to researching the issue outlined in the case, using actual evidence from the case where necessary. You should then point out the similarities and differences in relation to the research methods and data generated that would be created by the opposing philosophical approach, in a logical way.

- What is the opposing approach to knowledge construction?
- What types of methods are likely to be used by those subscribing to the opposing epistemology?
- What type of data and conclusions would using an opposing approach to knowledge construction (and its accompanying research methods) have produced?

Level 4: question the epistemological approach taken by the researchers

Use the following questions to help you make a recommendation (or not) in relation to the philosophical approach taken by the researchers, as outlined in the case. You should link this statement to underlying theory and provide actual evidence from the case scenario.

- How would a social scientist who believes in an opposing epistemology criticise the research outlined in the case?
- Which is the correct approach to the research in your opinion? How would you have set about examining the issue outlined in the background to the case?
- How would you justify your choice in light of others' assessment?

Concepts to consider

The following is a checklist of concepts to consider as you work through each case. The concepts relate directly to theory presented in Chapter 2 of this book. You are also urged to consider the contextualisation of the research cases in light of existing theory.

Some dos

- Consider the epistemological basis of the research – this should normally drive the research methodology, and ultimately the type of data generated.
- Consider whether the mechanism of research is in line with the epistemological position, for example:

  o Within the empirical framework, do the methods ensure objectivity; is there a clear hypothesis relating to finite variables; has inferential statistics been used; and are the outcomes generalisable?

  o With the interpretivist approach, what is the method of interpretation being used, e.g., grounded theory, thematic analysis or discourse analysis, and does the case meet the basic conventions of these methods?

Some don'ts

- Don't read the cases as anything but unsatisfactory. They are hypothetical and have been written to challenge readers' assumptions about what is acceptable research.
- Don't forget to consider if the data collection methods are appropriate and whether the correct type of data has been generated according to the epistemological position.
- Don't overlook the novelty aspect of the research – has anything original and new been established through the work? How are the results linked in with existing theory in the discussion section?
- Don't ignore the background section – in what way has the established theory from the preceding chapters of this book (or other recognised theory) been used to justify the work?
- Don't forget, a good paper quotes established theory as part of its background and discussion, not just the outcome of other research – so it will not suffice for the authors to merely quote other related work if existing theory can be cited.

Cases involving practice research

Anticoagulant counselling

Background: A baseline study of anticoagulant management in UK hospitals before the introduction of National Patient Safety Agency (NPSA) Alert 18 found significant problems with warfarin management across a large number of trusts, with 50% of consultant haematologists expressing concern about the discharge of patients on anticoagulants from general inpatient wards. We had anecdotal evidence that warfarin counselling at discharge needed to be improved at our hospital. A perception existed that patients discharged from the hospital were being readmitted because of warfarin-related morbidity with anecdotal evidence that those returning to anticoagulant clinics one week later had varied knowledge of their treatment, the dosing, potential side-effects, interactions, and other vital information. Yet, the specific problem we faced at the trust was an inability to highlight the problem in the absence of concrete and convincing evidence of process failures.

Aim and objectives: The challenge concerned not only a need to implement the recommendations in NPSA Alert 18 but also the need to assess, define and confirm a suspicion through appropriate methodology to justify a formal examination of the problem.

Methods: This work was conducted within one hospital trust in England. The focus was the safety of patients discharged from secondary care with warfarin, in line with NPSA Alert 18 *'Actions that Can Make Anticoagulant*

Therapy Safer. This work was conducted via methods that involved observations at ward level and an audit of patient knowledge at anticoagulant clinics. Appropriate ethical exemption was granted at the outset. Observations at ward level were conducted by a junior researcher and involved a prospective examination of warfarin counselling at discharge ($n = 17$) against a pre-designed template of ideal counselling points. Data collection at anticoagulant clinics ($n = 12$) involved a prospective review of patient knowledge by the clinic's nurse counsellors.

Results: The single most definitive outcome of the work was the assessment of and the ability to express the problem more definitively to justify a strategy for change. None of the patients observed at ward level received the full information at discharge with 15/17 receiving no information about the importance of INR measurements, 14 receiving no information about the management of bruising or bleeding and only 1 receiving information relating to potential warfarin interactions. At anticoagulant visits, only 7/12 patients knew the different-coloured tablets were of different strengths and only two knew about possible management of side-effects.

Discussion: Previous research had found some confusion between nurses, junior doctors and clinical pharmacists about the responsibility for completing the 'yellow book' (detailing anticoagulant-related information) on discharge. Unsafe arrangements and communications at discharge from hospital are known risk factors with anticoagulant therapy. In cash-strapped times, what we have learnt is the challenge of unearthing initial evidence of unsafe practices, to convince colleagues of the need for investment in formal and directed risk assessment of warfarin counselling for enhanced patient safety.

Conclusion: Although NPSA Alert 18 highlights action for making anticoagulant therapy safer, it may not tackle the sensitive issue of investigating and unearthing initial evidence of unsafe practices, which requires careful handling to ensure that all colleagues concur on the need for change.

Prescribing antipsychotics in dementia

Background: Dementia is primarily associated with a decline in cognitive function, but can also lead to behavioural changes that manifest as aggression and violence. While antipsychotics have been used to manage the behavioural and psychological symptoms of dementia (BPSD) their use is mainly off-licence because of lack of safety and effectiveness data. Antipsychotics in dementia can lead to an increased risk of death, including increased risk of a cerebrovascular event. In 2006, guidance on dementia from the National Institute for Health and Clinical Excellence (NICE) recommended using antipsychotics only in severe cases and once a number of conditions had been met. A later review by Professor Banerjee stated that although approximately 180 000 patients with dementia receive antipsychotics every year in the UK, only 36 000 may actually benefit. Yet antipsychotics continue to be used excessively and not in accordance with NICE recommendations.

Aim and objectives: One way in which practice can be improved is through research that examines current use. The purpose of this project was to conduct an examination of antipsychotic prescribing in patients with dementia at a mental health NHS trust.

Methods: Ethical approval was sought and gained. The patient population was chosen in accordance with NICE guidelines and the aim of the project was as follows: patients (of any age) with Alzheimer's disease, vascular dementia, mixed dementias or dementia with Lewy bodies with severe non-cognitive symptoms due to their dementia; patients prescribed antipsychotics for their non-cognitive symptoms (BPSD); and patients admitted to the hospital within a three-month period. For each patient, data were collected in relation to: whether active consent for treatment with antipsychotics had been sought; whether changes in cognition had been assessed and recorded afterwards; whether target symptoms had been identified and documented and subsequently tracked; whether a risk–benefit analysis had been conducted in relation to the choice of antipsychotic; whether the starting dose was low; and whether treatment had been time-limited and subject to regular review. Data were analysed descriptively.

Results: A total of 50 patients were eligible for inclusion. In 26 of 50 cases, there was no evidence of a full discussion about the possible risks and benefits of treatment. All patients had target symptoms identified and changes in cognition were assessed for all but one patient. Titrating the dose from a low dose to a higher dose had been carried out in all but four patients, who were given an initial higher dose of antipsychotic than recommended. Most patients had been given the option to undergo concomitant non-pharmacological treatment, such as art and craft workshops, reminiscence therapy, pottery making, games, music therapy and singing.

Discussion: Currently around 180 000 people with dementia are being treated with an antipsychotic drug. Many carers and relatives would argue that BPSD is the most important feature of dementia, contributing to caregiver burden and stress. Antipsychotics are frequently used to treat non-cognitive symptoms such as aggression and agitation, as well as hallucinations and delusions. According to NICE dementia guidelines, they should only be considered as first-line treatment if the patient is severely distressed or there is an immediate risk of harm to themselves or others. The current study found most patients had been prescribed an antipsychotic in accordance with the recommendations made by NICE.

Conclusion: NICE guidance was being adhered to in the main and there was no evidence of over-prescribing of antipsychotics in patients with BPSD.

Medicines Use Review service

Background: A Medicines Use Review (MUR) is an advanced service offered by community pharmacies as part of the current contractual agreement with the NHS in the UK. The aim of the service, in essence a private consultation, is to improve patient knowledge, concordance and use of medicines. While general practitioner and pharmacist views about the MUR have been investigated through formal research, lay perceptions about the service remain largely unknown.

Aim and objectives: Our objective was to test perceptions about who *should* conduct reviews relating to medicines. We used an experimental design and bespoke vignettes that relayed the same basic information to test our hypothesis that the general public would favour doctors in such a role compared with pharmacists. We tested another hypothesis that people would prefer review discussions to be focused on improving knowledge of medicine rather than actual medicines usage.

Methods: We designed a two-factor experiment using a hypothetical scenario about a patient on multiple medicines visiting either the doctor or the pharmacist for a discussion about their medication. Volunteer participants from the town centre were allocated at random to receive one of four scenarios all with the same basic information, but either with the doctor or the pharmacist being consulted, and also either with the focus of the consultation being improvement of knowledge or improvement of medicines usage. All participants received a questionnaire containing the scenario and the outcome measures on a 10-point Likert scale, including questions about perceived value of the service. Thirty participants received the doctor scenario and 30 the pharmacist scenario. Within each group, half received the knowledge-improvement scenario and the other half received the improved medicine-usage scenario. The project was approved by an ethics committee. Data from questionnaires were transferred to the statistical software SPSS and analysed using analysis of variance (ANOVA) with questions relating to the perceived value of the service as dependent variables. The category of health professional and aim of the service were independent variables.

Results: ANOVA showed a significant effect of 'service aim' on perceived service value, $F(4, 55) = 11.53, p < 0.005$, with those told the aim was only to improve knowledge giving higher 'value of service' ratings (mean of three questions relating to perceived value). ANOVA also showed a significant effect of category of health professional, $F(4, 55) = 7.28, p < 0.05$, on perceived value, with those presented with the doctor scenario giving higher ratings.

Discussion: Giving information about the aim of a 'review of medicines' service affected perceptions of the worth of such as service. Participants also gave higher ratings of value when they were told that the doctor would be conducting the review. Presumably people use information relating to both the aim of a service as well as who is conducting it to judge the value of a medicines review service. We could argue that although the public still valued the role a pharmacist might play in medicines reviews, they did nonetheless consider such a service provided by the doctor as being more valuable.

Conclusion: Given the option, the general public prefer doctors to conduct medicines reviews and prefer the focus of such reviews to be the improvement of knowledge about medicines. This brings into question the value of the pharmacy MUR to the general public.

Antidepressants and adherence

Background: Depression is thought to affect around 15% of populations worldwide. It is a disease that can disrupt daily activity and work and even lead to death through suicide. Although the pharmacological treatment of depression involves taking antidepressant medication, a large number of patients do not currently receive any form of treatment for depression. Among those who do receive treatment, only 50% are thought to adhere to their antidepressant regimen. One of the reasons that patients may stop taking antidepressants relates to perceptions about the safety and effectiveness of these medicines in treating depression. Newspaper discourse has been shown to be responsible for influencing both public perceptions and behaviour in a number of health-related domains. We wanted to investigate the role of the UK press in constructing normative knowledge about antidepressant medication.

Aim and objectives: The aim was to investigate the social construction of knowledge about antidepressant medication by UK broadsheet and tabloid newspapers using discourse analysis. The primary objective was to analyse the discourse used to identify linguistic and descriptive patterns contributing to the portrayal of antidepressants.

Methods: We included four broadsheet and four tabloid newspapers in the search and retrieved all published articles relating to antidepressants for the period January 2007 to December 2009, inclusive. Discourse analysis was employed by three investigators to examine the way language and imagery had been used to symbolise and give meaning to antidepressant medication, especially the portrayal of its side-effects and the role of the pharmaceutical industry in promoting antidepressant use. Special consideration was given to the way in which the patient, the doctor and the pharmaceutical industry were portrayed, and implied power relations.

Results: A total of 1125 newspaper articles were analysed, 44.7% from UK broadsheets ($n = 503$) and 55.3% from UK tabloids ($n = 622$). A total of 957 articles (85%) were primarily focused on the side-effects of antidepressants. Only a minority of the articles focused on the role of the pharmaceutical industry in promoting antidepressants. The potential for antidepressants to cause addiction, side-effects and worsening of general health overshadowed discussions about potential benefits of antidepressant therapy.

Discussion: We wanted to examine the social construction of antidepressants by the UK press. We found a variety of language had been used to describe antidepressants, which overall did not portray these medicines as beneficial or even effective. Although the articles did not focus on the role of the pharmaceutical industry in promoting antidepressant medication, as had been thought originally, there was nonetheless a focus on the role of doctors in over-promoting antidepressant usage. If patient adherence to medication is to be addressed, it is important to recognise and understand the role that the media play in forming perceptions about medication. Headlines such as 'Antidepressants made my life hell' and 'Withdrawal from antidepressants is depressing' are unhelpful to health professionals who are attempting to deal with low adherence rates.

Conclusion: Pharmacists are ideally placed to interact with patients and to reform perceptions relating to medication. Making pharmacists aware of media representations could be a first move in changing the social construction of antidepressants as harmful medicines.

New Medicine Service

Background: The New Medicine Service (NMS) was the fourth advanced service to be introduced into the UK NHS community pharmacy contract. The service was implemented in late 2011. Its aim is to support medicines adherence in those patients who have been newly prescribed a medicine for a chronic condition. Patients with asthma, chronic obstructive pulmonary disease, type 2 diabetes, prescribed anticoagulant/antiplatelet therapy or with hypertension were included in the initial rollout of the NMS. Although the Medicines Use Review (MUR) service, another 'cognitive pharmacy service', had been introduced six years earlier, there was no convincing evidence of its effect on improving patient adherence to medicines. We wanted to gauge perceptions about the ability of the NMS to improve adherence where the MUR had 'failed'.

Aim and objectives: The aim was to interview pharmacists to establish views relating to the NMS, specifically its potential to improve patient adherence.

Methods: A total of 32 pharmacist participants were involved in the study. We recruited 12 participants to two focus group interviews ($n = 5$ and $n = 7$) and additionally conducted face-to-face interviews with 20 participants, all of whom were interviewed by the same researcher. Grounded theory was used to analyse all interview transcripts, transferred to N-Vivo, to generate a model relating to perceptions about the NMS. The model is based around competencies and patient expectations and brings a rich understanding of pharmacists' cynicism and confidence in relation to the new service. Ethical approval was obtained in advance.

Results: Two general types of perception can be associated with the provision of 'cognitive pharmacy services' such as the NMS. The first represents a strong negative perception of pharmacists' own competence to conduct consultation-type services and can be sourced back to experiences with the MUR. The real barrier here appears to be linked to a lack of external recognition of pharmacists' worth and contribution to improving patient health through the MUR. This type of thinking leads to a reluctant and unwelcome acceptance of the changing role of the pharmacist. It also leads to a form of disassociation with the aims of the service, where pharmacists accept their role but only as providers of a service whose ultimate outcome cannot be foreseen. The second perception centres on patient expectations. A small minority of pharmacists, who are generally more altruistic in their attitude to work and optimistic about the profession as a whole, see their ultimate professional objective as one of 'service provision' to meet patient expectations. Although at first glance this category is focused on provision of a service, in wanting to meet patient expectations, these pharmacists accepted their role and therefore ability to improve patient adherence through the NMS.

Discussion: If the NMS is to succeed, lessons must be learnt from the MUR experience. A dynamic model was developed to map out and bring a more complete understanding of pharmacists' ideas about their ability to influence adherence through cognitive services such as the MUR and the NMS. Two predominant attitudes existed. Although it could be argued that there was some evidence of optimism and willingness to fully engage in an adherence-improving service, this category of attitude existed only in a small proportion of the participants interviewed. The overall scepticism that was unearthed has to be tackled systematically if the NMS is to succeed as a service that helps improve adherence.

Conclusion: A model has been constructed to explain the prevailing attitudes of pharmacists towards cognitive pharmacy services such as the NMS and could be used as a basis for engaging with pharmacists to help improve chances of a successful new advanced service.

Glossary

Actor/observe effect

A type of cognitive bias where people tend to select external attributions to explain their own behaviour.

Adherence (supersedes the term compliance)

The extent to which the patient's behaviour matches agreed recommendations from the prescriber. With intentional non-adherence, the patient has decided not to follow the recommendations, whereas with unintentional non-adherence, the patient either forgets or, for example, has problems with the packaging.

Anchoring and adjustment heuristic

A decision-making strategy that operates when people estimate the answer to a question based on an initial value presented to them as part of the question.

Appraisal (theory)

The notion that cognitive appraisal of a stimulus takes place before the experience of emotion takes place.

Atomism

An approach to research which asserts that objects of scientific study are interpretable through analysis into distinct and discrete elementary components.

Attribution theory

Description of people's perception and explanation of their social environment, specifically in relation to the reasons they give for other people's behaviour in the form of feelings, beliefs and intentions.

Audit

Collecting data to compare practice with defined standards.

Availability heuristic	A decision-making strategy that operates when people predict the likelihood of something by the ease with which similar instances can be recalled.
Base-rate fallacy	Cognitive bias involving the failure to take account of the prior probability of an event when making a judgement.
Biomedical model of health	A biological and medicinal conceptualisation of health.
Bio-psychosocial model of health	The conceptualisation of health as an interaction between biological/medical, psychological and social determinants.
Body language	Communicating non-verbally through movement or conduct of the body including the face.
Categorical variable	Characterised by independent and separate data groups.
Causal law	Where one variable is shown to cause an effect in the other through scientific law.
Chronic disease	Illnesses that are prolonged, do not resolve spontaneously, and are rarely cured completely.
Closed systems in research	Where a limited number of measurable variables are involved, to the exclusion of others to avoid confounding, so that clear relationships between the variables can be predicted.
Cognition	Mental processes occurring in the mind of an individual.
Cognitive behaviour therapy	A form of therapy that attempts to correct misaligned thoughts and to alter unwanted behaviours and mental health disorders.
Cognitive biases in decision making	Inaccurate judgements that occur due to the use of heuristics.
Cognitive models	Schematic representations that help psychologists predict mental processes.
Cognitive pharmacy	The use of cognitive psychology to understand pharmacy-related thoughts and beliefs.
Cognitive pharmacy service	The use of cognitive psychology in a structured attempt to change patients' behaviour through the practice of pharmacy.

Cognitive restructuring	Using specific techniques to alter the pattern of thinking.
Common-sense model of self-regulation	A model related to conceptualisation and management of illness by individuals, whereby cognitive and emotional representations of the health threat direct the coping mechanism, and where a secondary appraisal and consequent changes all characterise the patient's attempt to self-regulate the illness.
Compliance	*See* Adherence.
Concordance	A consultation process which involves the prescriber and the patient coming to an agreed therapeutic decision but the term can also define patient support in medicine taking as well as prescribing communication.
Confidence interval	The likely estimate within which the population mean falls (for example the 95% confidence), based on the mean and standard error from the sample.
Confounding	A variable that has not been controlled for and which then interferes with the findings of a study.
Conjunction fallacy	Cognitive bias whereby a combination of two or more attributes is judged more probable than either attribute on its own.
Constant comparison	In an analytical process such as grounded theory, this involves regularly checking the categories that emerge against the data to enable readjustment as needed.
Continuous variable	Characterised by data that can fall anywhere along a scale.
Discourse analysis	A qualitative method of analysing interactive speech.
Emergent theory	In research such as grounded theory, this refers to theory arising from the data as ideas are put together, and which itself might direct further data collection and analysis.
Emotional intelligence	The ability to perceive emotions correctly and to use emotions and emotional knowledge to enhance thought.

Empiricism	A theory of knowledge based around experience and evidence where discoveries are made through testable quantitative research.
Epistemology	The theory of knowledge relating to how we know what we know.
Ethnographic	A methodological approach that involves researchers immersing themselves in a social setting so as to report back from the perspective of the setting's members.
Expectancy	*See* Value-expectancy theory.
Experiments	A method of research that enables the manipulation of a set of variables to observe and measure their impact on other variables.
Facts	Objective, observable truths.
Framing effect	Cognitive bias that describes the impact that the explanation, labelling, or arrangement of a problem can have on responses to the problem.
Fundamental attribution error	A type of bias where people tend to explain the behaviour of others by using internal attributions.
Fuzzy trace theory	A model relating to health decision-making which states that people prefer to use gist representations of information, integrating them with their values, principles and knowledge, before making judgements and decisions.
Grounded theory	An inductive process of analysis that derives theory from the data, so that theory is 'grounded' in the qualitative data from which it is developed.
Health-damaging (risky) behaviours	Behaviours associated with increased susceptibility to a specific cause of ill health.
Health belief model	A model relating to people's health-related beliefs and behaviours, the core constructs of which are perceived susceptibility, perceived severity, perceived benefits and perceived barriers, cues to action, and a later addition of self-efficacy.
Health inequities	The unfair and avoidable differences in health status seen within and between countries.

Health psychology	The use of psychology to understand psychological aspects of health promotion, disease prevention, treatment and identification of psychological causes and patterns of health and illness.
Healthy behaviours	Any activity undertaken by an individual for the purpose of promoting, protecting or maintaining health, regardless of its effectiveness.
Heuristics	Strategies based on readily available mental representations of the world, which can be evoked during decision making to make the process faster.
Hypothesis	Proposed, precise explanation for the relationship between a set of variables.
Idiographic	Research methods that attempt to study unique individuals or persons.
Inductive	A process of analysing qualitative data that enables theory or concepts to be derived from the data rather than from preformed hypotheses.
Integrative model of behavioural change	*See* Reasoned action approach.
Intentional non-adherence	*See* Adherence.
Interactional model	*See* Transactional model of stress and coping.
Interpretation	A theory of knowledge based around the analysis of meaning in subjective accounts through qualitative research.
Mean	The arithmetic mean of a set of data is the average value obtained by adding up the total scores and dividing by the sample number, to give the central tendency of the data.
Medical psychology	The use of psychology to understand problems that arise in medicine including psychological aspects of pain, terminal illness, bereavement, disability and reactions to medical advice.

Medical sociology	The use of sociological knowledge to aid diagnosis, treatment, teaching and research in medicine.
Methodology	The concept underlying a set of methods.
Methods	Systematic detail of a research procedure.
Naturalism	The belief that the methods of the natural sciences can be transferred to the study of humans.
Nominalism	An approach to research that asserts concepts not directly experienced through the senses are meaningless.
Nomothetic	Research methods that attempt to create general, scientific laws.
Non-adherence	*See* Adherence.
Normal distribution	The pattern of values typified by a Gaussian, bell-shaped, symmetrical (about its mid-point) curve, that is assumed for parametric tests.
Normative theories in decision making	Concerned with making the ideal decision and what ought to happen in a perfect model.
Null hypothesis	The assumption that there is no relationship between the variables being studied in research.
Objective	Free of bias or prejudice.
Occupational health psychology	The use of psychology to understand and improve the quality of people's work and the protection and promotion of the health, safety and well-being of those at work.
Ontology	The theory of the nature of existence or what it is to be human
Open system of research	Where complexity is acknowledged, no real external boundary is assumed and multiple causal relationships cannot be predicted with accuracy.
Operationalising	Bringing the research ideas into fruition through a pragmatic approach.

Overconfidence bias	Cognitive bias whereby people's expressions of confidence in the accuracy of their own judgements are largely unreliable resulting in higher confidence ratings when measured against actual correctness.
Parametric tests	Branch of statistics that assumes data satisfy certain population parameters, for example are normally distributed.
Parsonian model	*See* Sick role.
Pharmaceutical psychology	The use of psychology to understand people's beliefs and behaviour in relation to the activities of the modern-day pharmacist.
Pharmaceutical sociology (social pharmacy)	The use of sociological knowledge as it relates to the work of the pharmacist.
Phenomenalism	An approach to research that asserts only knowledge gained through the physical senses exists.
Population	All possible group members of interest to the study, from which normally a sample is withdrawn for study.
Positivism	A philosophical position about knowledge creation that aims to create general laws that express relationships between observable variables.
Primacy debate (in relation to emotion)	A debate about whether cognition precedes emotion or vice versa.
Probability sampling	The random selection of a sample from the target population so that each individual has a known chance of being selected.
Psychology	The study of the human mind and its functions as it relates to human behaviour, cognition (thought) and experience.
Purposive sampling	The selection of a sample from the target population based on the characteristics of the participants rather than selection at random.
Qualitative research	Research methods, informed by interpretative epistemology, that attempt to bring meaning and create an understanding of humans.

Quantitative research	Research methods, informed by positivist epistemology, that attempt to use measurements to produce numerical relationships.
Rationality	The ability to use reason to make decisions.
Reasoned action approach	Includes the theory of reasoned action and the theory of planned behaviour – a health behaviour model with seven major constructs of intention, attitude, perceived norms, self-efficacy or perceived behavioural control, behavioural beliefs, normative beliefs and control beliefs.
Reductionism	An approach to studying phenomena that reduces the object of study down to its component parts.
Reflexive	In qualitative research this refers to the researcher's acknowledgement of how their own experiences/attitudes may have influenced their interpretation of the data and therefore the study conclusions.
Regression fallacy	Cognitive bias whereby natural regression towards the mean is interpreted as attributable to something other than chance.
Reliability	The extent to which the same results can be achieved over time and comparable conditions.
Replicable	In research, this refers to the ability to reproduce the same results every time.
Representative	In the context of research, this is the type of sample that allows generalisations to be made about the population under study.
Representativeness heuristic	A decision-making strategy that operates when people categorise things/events by considering their similarity to the group/category.
Research	The systematic investigation into and study of materials and sources in order to establish facts and reach new conclusions.
Research ethics	The application of ethical principles for the protection of research participants, researchers, and ultimately science and society.
Research hypothesis	*See* Hypothesis.

Research question	The focus of the investigation in terms of answers sought.
Sample	A subset of the population selected for study.
Sample size	The number of participants making up the sample selected for research.
Sample-size fallacy	A cognitive bias whereby the sample size is not taken into account when estimating the probability of obtaining a value in a sample obtained from a population.
Sampling error	The difference between data produced from the sample and data that might have been produced had it been possible to take measurements from the entire population.
Schemata	Generalised mental representations of social phenomena based on shared (social) knowledge about an array of matters such as people, events, roles, objects akin to stereotypes.
Scientific law	A formal statement about a quantifiable, definitive causal relationship between the stated variables.
Self-efficacy (in relation to behaviour)	An individual's personal conviction about their ability to change their behaviour (or a similar challenge) in light of their own beliefs and circumstances.
Self-regulation theory	*See* Common-sense model of self-regulation.
Self-serving bias	Relating to causal attributions, describes a bias where successes are related to internal causes and failures to external ones.
Sick role	A concept put forward by Talcott Parsons relating to social expectations about being sick (accepted as ill).
Social and cognitive pharmacy	The application of both sociology and cognitive psychology in pharmacy.
Social cognition	The mental processing of social knowledge.

Social cognitive theory	A health behaviour theory that asserts behaviour is determined by expectancies and incentives, with core constructs of knowledge, perceived self-efficacy, outcome expectations, health goals, and perceived facilitators and impediments to change.
Social determinants of health	The structural determinants and conditions of daily life that determine people's chances of leading a healthy and flourishing life.
Social institution	Social practices that are sanctioned and maintained by social norms.
Social pharmacy	*See* Pharmaceutical sociology.
Social psychology	The psychology of social interactions.
Society	A collection of people sharing common traditions, institutions, territories, activities and interests.
Sociology	The scientific study of society.
Stages-of-change model	*See* Transtheoretical model.
Stimulus response	A theory of learning according to which behaviour is determined by its consequences.
Standard deviation	A measure of the dispersion of data about the mean. For data that are normally distributed, about 95% of individuals will have values within two standard deviations of the mean.
Standard error	This is calculated by dividing the standard deviation by the square root of the sample size and tends to fall as the sample size increases.
Subjective	Seen from the personal perspective of the subject.
Surveys	A method of research that attempts to collect information systematically using a questionnaire as the basis.
Thematic analysis	Categorising qualitative data into themes and not necessarily to form new theory.
Themes	In qualitative research, summaries of findings from the text.

Theoretical saturation	In analytical processes such as grounded theory, this is the point beyond which no new categories emerge and further modification of the theory is inconsequential.
Theory	An idea or proposition about something.
Theory of planned behaviour	*See* Reasoned action approach.
Theory of reasoned action	*See* Reasoned action approach.
Transactional model of stress and coping	A cognitive model based on primary and secondary appraisals of stressors, which emphasises that stress occurs when coping resources and responses are outweighed by the demands of the stressor.
Transtheoretical model	A behavioural change model that has 'stages of change' at its core and considers change as progressing through stages of change including precontemplation, contemplation, preparation, action, maintenance and finally termination.
Unintentional non-adherence	*See* Adherence.
Validity	The extent to which what is being measured is genuine.
Value-expectancy theory	Predicts behaviour as a function of the subjective value of an outcome and the subjective probability (expectation) that such an outcome will be achieved as a result of the behaviour.
Values	People's subjective moral principles.
Variables	The attributes of an object of study being measured.

Index